Grandmasters of China ™

Volume One

Traditional Chinese Kungfu Series

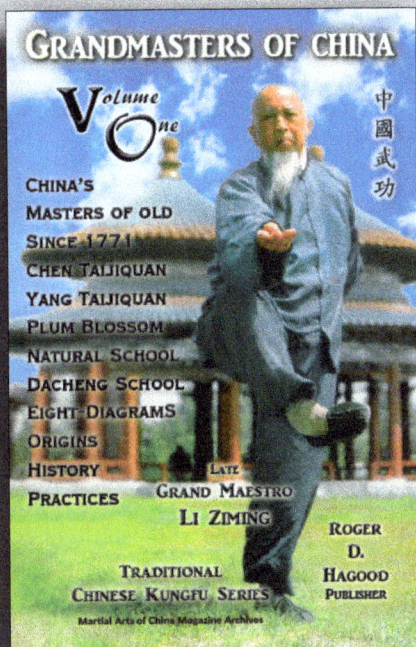

Publisher
Roger D. Hagood

Editors
Charles Alan Clemens
Patrick M. Wright

Southern Mantis Press | Pingshan Town, China

Southern Mantis Press
462 W. Virginia St. (Rt. 14)
Crystal Lake, Illinois 60014
1-800-Jook Lum
books@southernmantispress.com

Ordering Information:
Special discounts are available for martial art schools, bookstores, specialty shops, museums and events. Contact the publisher at the address above.

Original publication copyright © 1990 by China Direct Publishing, Inc. Roger D. Hagood, Publisher.

Cover photograph: Grandmaster Li Ziming, before his passing, had personally taught the Eight-Diagrams Palm School to more than 1,000 students. He was instrumental in opening more than 21 schools in Beijing alone. Story on page 73.

ISBN: 978-0-9857240-5-4

Traditional Chinese Kungfu Series

Grandmasters Of China

Volume One

Southern Mantis Press | Pingshan Town, China

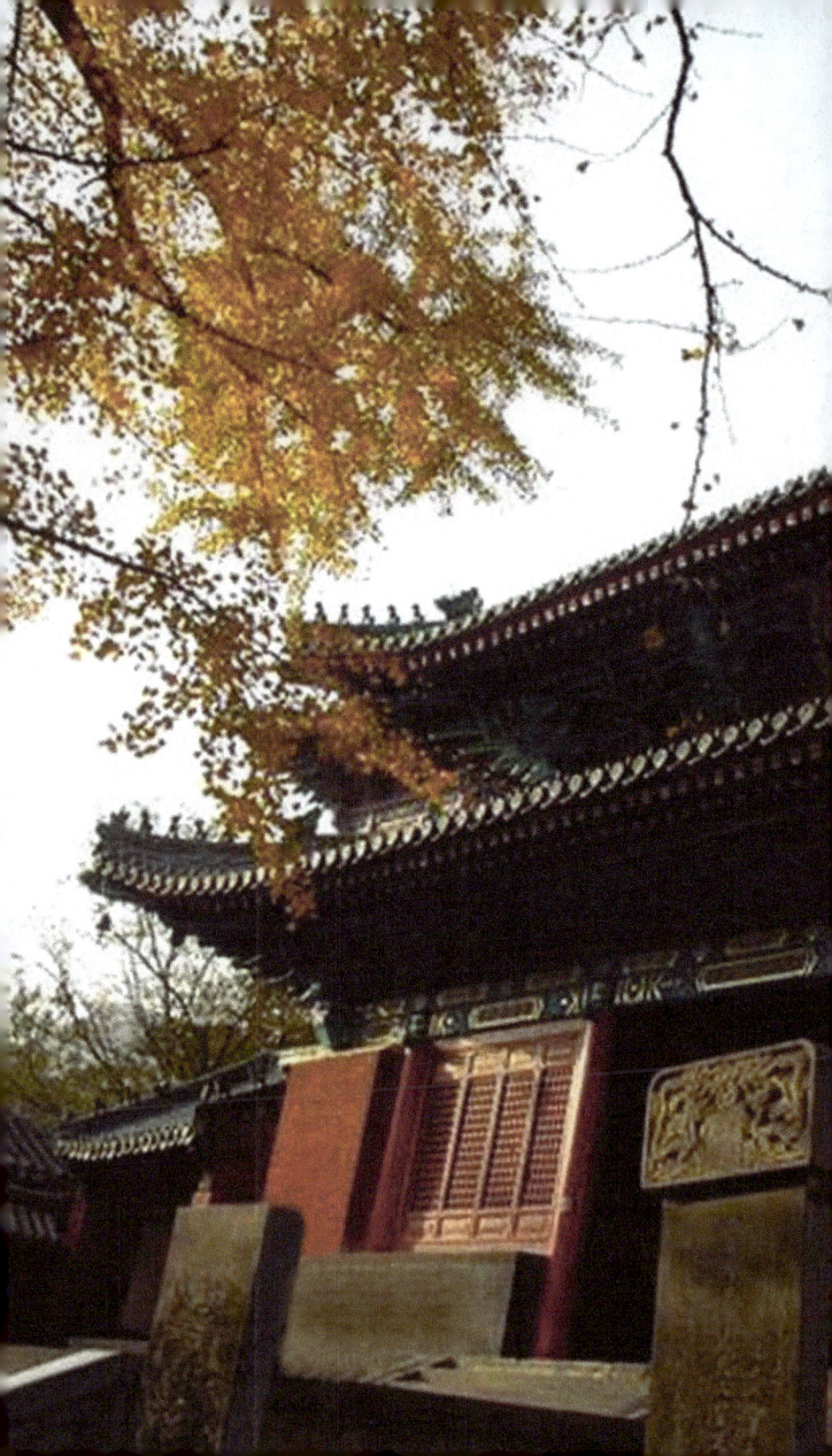

SHAOLIN TEMPLE

少林寺

Henan Province, China

Home of
External Work

It is said that the Shaolin School of boxing was inspired by the Indian Monk, Bodhidharma, circa 530 CE.

Six Externals

- **FISTS:** straight line attacks; circular defense

- **EYES:** eyes to eyes

- **ARMS:** crooked but not, straight but not, rolling in and out

- **STEPS:** solid, steady, heavy, light, agile within the space of a lying cow

- **BODY:** natural in up, down, left, right, forward

- **STRENGTH:** Hard strength mixed with gentleness to achieve the natural

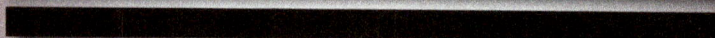

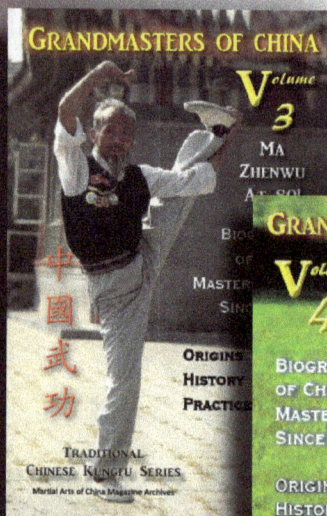

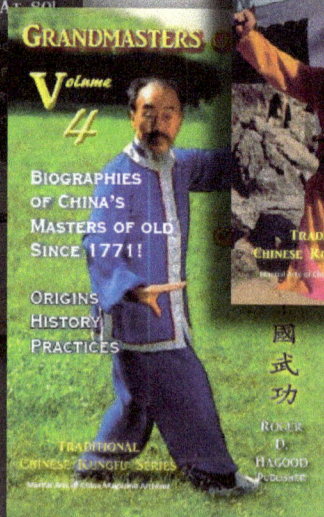

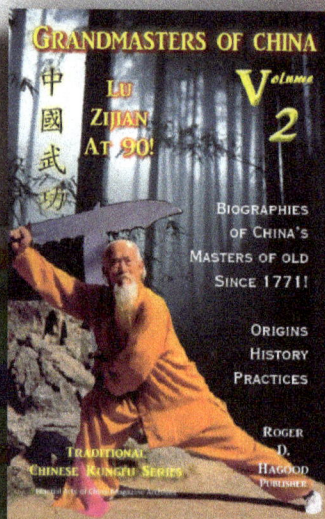

Dedication

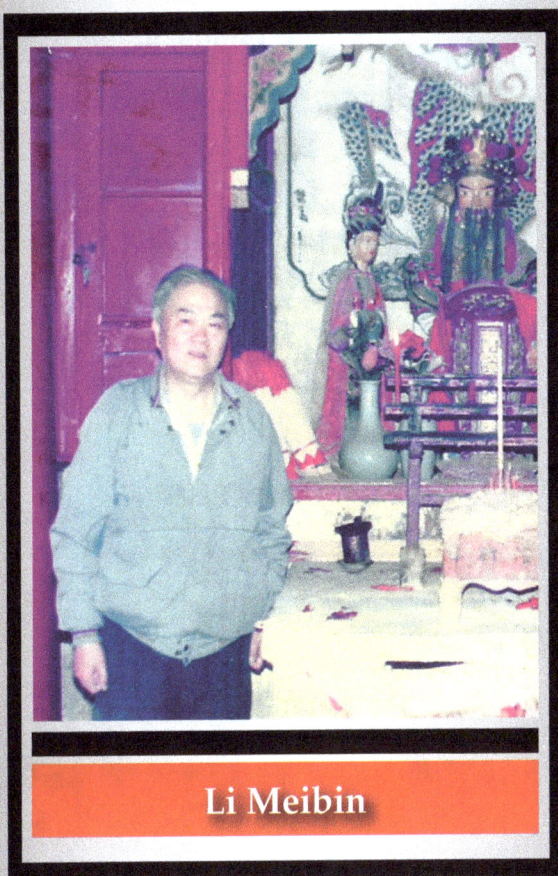

Li Meibin

Mr. Li Meibin was one of those few chosen by the Chinese authorities to attend the University of Illinois, Chicago, in the 1930s. After graduation, he brought an American flair and perspective back to his homeland and worked in various capacities including editor of *China Sports* Magazine in Beijing. We travelled China extensively together in the late '80s and early '90s and I gained a unique understanding from his old-school Chinese culture and Americanized views. He was instrumental in my publishing *Martial Arts of China* Magazine and this *Grandmasters of China* book series. In the above photo, circa 1989, he and I were visiting the Dragon Wells of Longquan, where China's most famous swords are still cast today. Mr. Li knew the meaning of brother-friendship. Special thanks to him and all the *China Sports* staff.

Table of Contents

RDH: How This Book Was Written—And Why

I originally published this book series, *Grandmasters of China™*, as *Martial Arts of China* newsstand magazine from 1989 - 1991. This *Traditional Chinese Kungfu Series* is a fresh twist in book format of those original magazines. The information herein is timeless and just as pertinent for traditional martial artists today, as it ever was. To know the future one must search the past and this book series is an innovative probe into China's masters of old.

In the '80s, I was an avid reader and subscriber of *China Sports* Magazine published by the China State Sports Commission in Beijing. That magazine contained a section on martial arts in each issue. I was also writing articles for several USA martial arts magazines under a pseudonym. In fact, my *Inside Kungfu* magazine articles were awarded "Best of the Year" several times in the '80s.

Putting the two together, a sports magazine from China and my writing, I decided to contact *China Sports* in Beijing and propose a joint venture to create a traditional Chinese kungfu magazine direct from the source - mother China! The magazines were launched in 1989 and became collector's items in the early 90s. They were distributed on the newsstand in fifteen countries.

From 1983 - 1986, the Chinese government mobilized 8,000 field workers at national and local levels to travel to the remotest corners of China and survey some 15,000 old kungfu masters. It was determined there were some 130 distinct styles of Chinese boxing, each with its own distinctive origin, features, and principles. In addition to collecting old boxing manuals, ancient weapons, and wushu antiques, several hundred hours of videotape were collected. This book (series) and the *China National Kungfu Survey on Videotape™* is the result of that early effort of the Chinese government to preserve traditional martial arts.

Down through the ages, many of the traditional schools and branches have been intertwined and overlapped with one another. Though opinions may vary greatly from different angles or points of view, we are still able to draw some rough lines of demarcation among the various schools and styles by studying the life sketches of the founders of the major schools and their representative successors. Collect every volume of *Grandmasters of China* and the *China National Kungfu Survey on Videotape* and discover their legacy!

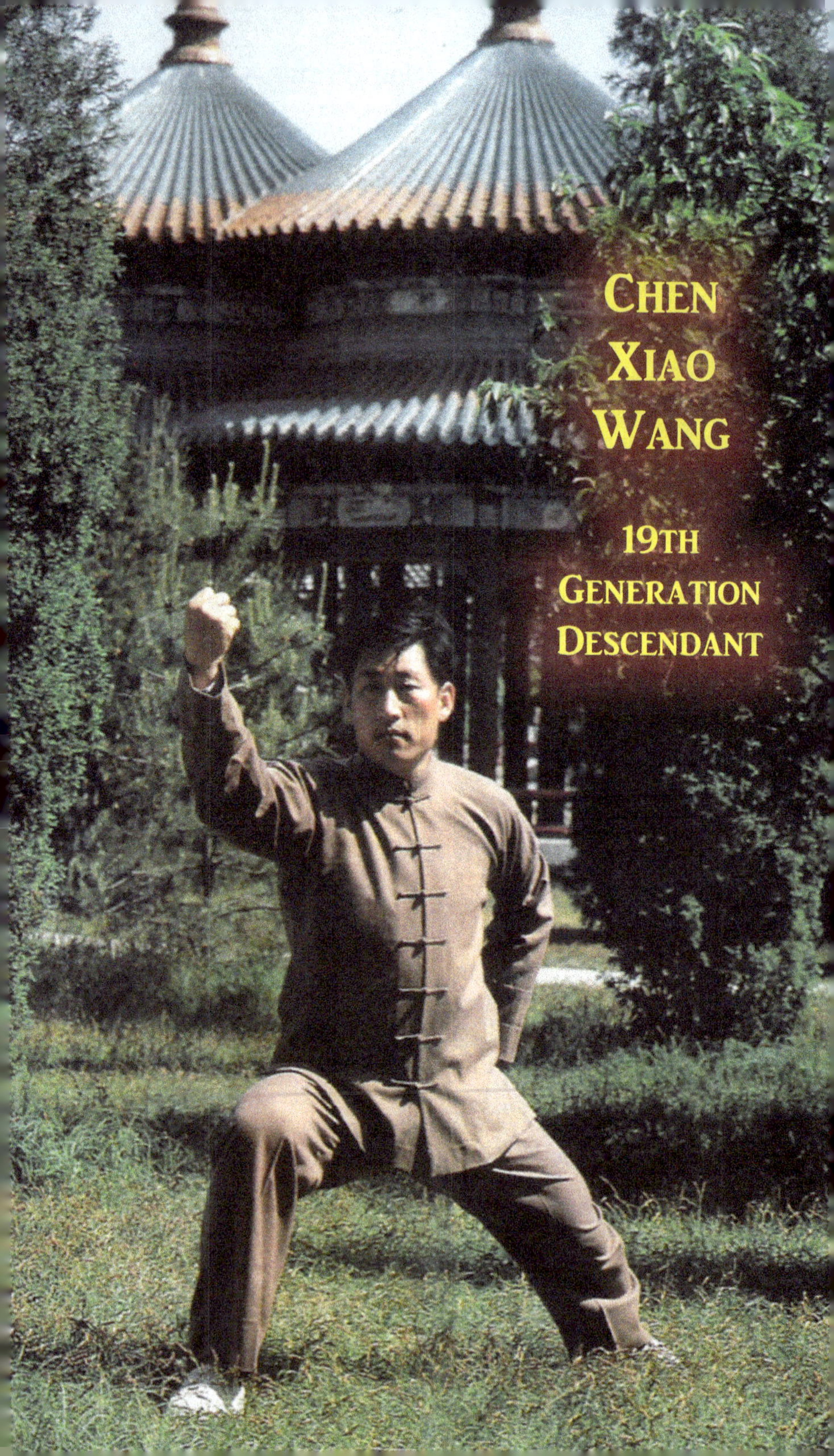

CHEN
XIAO
WANG

19TH
GENERATION
DESCENDANT

ABOUT

Chen-style

TAIJIQUAN

The Chen-style taijiquan is divided into two kinds of frames: old and new. Originally, the old frame consisted of five routines in 13 forms, in addition to a changquan (long-range boxing) routine in 108 forms and a set of paochui (cannon boxing) exercise.

From the period of Chen Changxing (1771-1853) and Chen Youben in the 19th century, the masters in Chenjiagou Village of Wenxian County in Henan Province concentrated on practising and perfecting their skills in taijiquan routine one, paochui routine one and tuishou (push-hands duet), all barehanded fighting techniques without any protector or equipment.

The old frame routine one now consists of 83 forms, with the following main characteristics:

(1) The movements are circular, rounded, or "spiral" with will-controlled force reaching the four extremities, that is, the tips of one's hands and feet, and with "external work" well coordinated with "internal work."

(2) There is an interaction and harmony between hardness and softness, with the inner force flowing deeply yet smoothly.

(3) Actions are regulated by respiration, circulation of qi, and exertion of force. Attention is concentrated on the dantian acupoint below the navel when qi sinks to that area. Exhalation is accompanied by utterances of such sounds as bi, si, xi or chui to increase explosive force.

(4) Quick movements are alternated swiftly with slow movements, which usually happen when the hands are moving in a circular path.

(5) The exercises can be performed in a high, middle or low body position, the high preferably by the aged and the weak and the low by young and strong people.

II The old frame routine two now consists of paochui in 71 forms, with the following main characteristics:

(1) The movements are faster, more forceful and more explosive than those of routine one.

(2) There are many energetic movements such as stamping, jumps and jerks, which are suitable for young and strong people, but are not so popular.

The new frame exists in two routines. One has a smaller frame and smaller circular movements than does the old and has some of the difficult parts removed. That's why people in Chenjiagou also refer to it as "small circle boxing" and to the old frame as "big circle boxing."

Above) "Thrice change palm" by Feng Dabiao, one of Chen Zhaokui's followers

Right) "Single Whip" by Chen Fake's grandson, Chen Yu

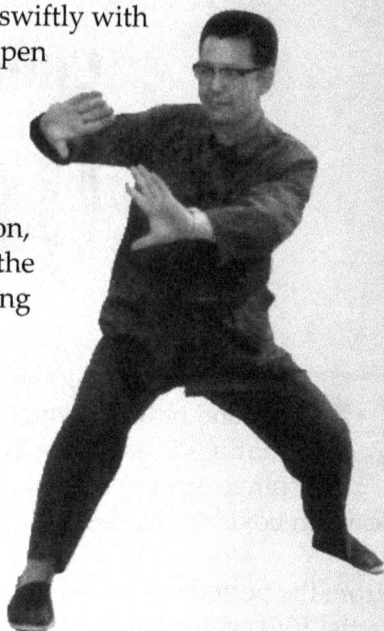

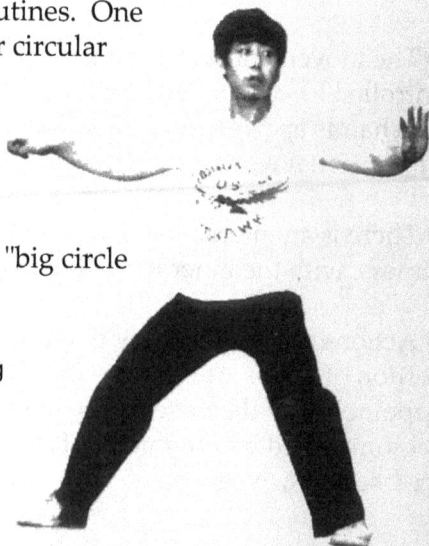

When the teaching was passed down to Chen Xin (1849-1929), the grandnephew of Chen Youben, it was summarized in his book, *The Illustrated Chen-Style Taijiquan*.

The other routine, arranged by Chen Youben's disciple Chen Qingping (1795-1868), is a small-frame exercise with slow, well-knit and complicated circular movements. It was passed on to others from Zhaobao Town of Wenxian County, so people call it "Zhaobao frame."

The Chen-style taijiquan is the oldest in China, on which all the other chief styles - Yang, Wu, Wu and Sun - are based.

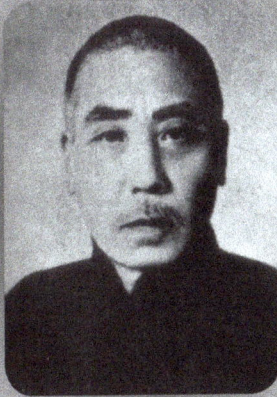

Chen Fake
(1887-1957)

A Worthy Successor to Chen-style Taijiquan

Chen Fake (pronounced Fa-Kuh) was a great-grandson of the great taijiquan master Chen Changxing and belonged to the 17th generation of the Chen family in Chenjiagou village, Henan, China.

Chen Fake was a sickly child and improved his health by practising taijiquan handed down from his forefathers. When he grew up, his interest in this art greatly increased. He would do the exercise 10 times in the morning, afternoon and evening, without a letup even in hot summer or severe winter.

Thanks to strict family guidance and his own effort, Chen Fake was a recognized taijiquan master when only 17. At 20, he beat a strong field of opponents in an open challenge and made a name for himself.

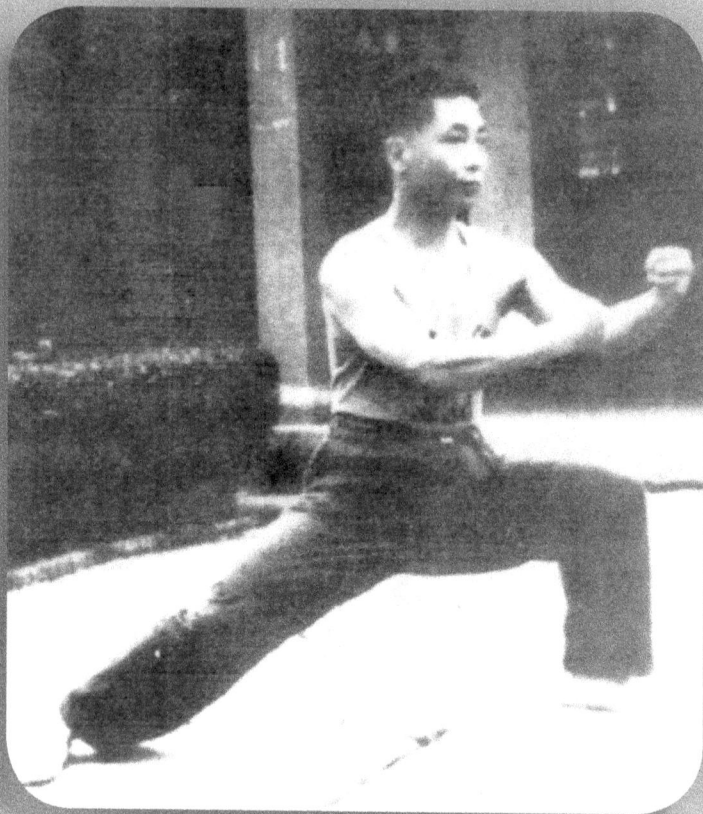

Chen Zhaokui (1928-1981), son of Chen Fake

In 1928, he came to Beijing at his nephew Chen Zhaopi's invitation. At that time, there were the notorious "three Li brothers" who played the bully everywhere in the city. One day, the two Chens came to the Lis' to teach them a lesson. Seeing nothing particular about them, the eldest Li haughtily stepped forward with a heavy punch. But before his fist could touch Chen Zhaopi's face Chen Fake darted forward and, with an angry cry, swept the attacker off his feet and threw him onto a windowsill. The incident soon became the talk of the town, and the name of Chen Fake became widely known, especially among the wushu circles.

As a growing number of people came to learn taijiquan out of admiration for him, Chen Fake set up the Zhongzhou Wushu Centre in Beijing's Xuanwumen District. Among the applicants were even skilled wushu masters including Liu Ruizhi, Tang Hao, Li Jingwu, Gu Liuxin and Feng Zhiqiang.

Chen Fake never had the chance to go to school, but he was an honest and tolerant person. His simplicity and uprightness won him great respect from his disciples. Once, a university invited him to be a wushu teacher, but when he learned the authorities were going to discharge the former one, he objected, insisting that they engage two wushu teachers at the same time, for he would never want others to lose their jobs because of him.

Although held in high esteem as a great taijiquan master, Chen Fake never belittled other schools. When his disciples asked him what kind of wushu was the best, his invariable answer was that all schools, taijiquan included, are good so long as they have survived the tests of time; otherwise they would have long been eliminated.

He believed that whether a school of wushu is good or bad depends to a large extent on the way of teaching and learning. At the beginning, it is the teacher who has the primary role to play and a good teacher should have a good knowledge of what he is teaching and he should be able to point out the correct way to learn for his students. As for who will learn faster, it all depends on the learners themselves. He also said that learning taijiquan is just like learning calligraphy. For instance, most people know Wang Xizhi as a great calligrapher in the Jin Dynasty (265-420), but Yan Zhenqing, Liu Gongquan and Ouyang Xun of the Tang Dynasty (618-907), and Zhao Mengfu of the Song Dynasty (960-1279) were also great calligraphers with their own styles. One might like Wang's calligraphy better and learn from him, but one could not say that the other four masters' calligraphy was not good and of no value. Chen's words have been taken by his followers as a maxim that one should always be modest and draw on the strong points of different schools.

After the founding of the People's Republic in 1949, Chen Fake set up the Capital Wushu Society together with Hu Yaozhen and continued teaching the Chen-style taijiquan. In 1953, he and three other famous taijiquan masters Wang Xialin, Deng Hongzao and Ma Xichun represented North China in the First National Wushu Competition in Tianjin. Having taught wushu in Beijing for nearly three decades, Chen Fake had pupils everyhere in and outside China. Many of them are carrying on their master's cause to spread the Chen-style taijiquan even today.

Anecdotes of Chen Fake

A challenge contest was going to take place in Beijing. Chen Fake was invited by its supervisor to be a consultant. At a meeting to discuss the rules, some people proposed that every bout last 15 minutes. Chen said that the duration would be too long and the contest would be protracted with so many entrants. Besides, he added, even an ordinary fight in the street would take only a few seconds to decide the outcome, sometimes even before you have counted up to three.

"Really?" said Li Zhaohua, a six-footer teaching wushu at the Northeast University.

"Let's have a trial bout and everything will be clear," replied Chen with a smile.

Li charged forward with a push, Chen side-stepped it at a lightning speed and counter-attacked with but a slight force of his elbow. Li bumped against the wall and a photo frame fell from it and broke into pieces. "Now I believe what you say," he murmured. "But you've almost frightened my soul out!"

"You don't have to worry," Chen assured him. "I won't hurt anybody."

Sure enough, Li felt no pain when he touched all over his body, although the fabric of his jacket was rubbed in with some lime powder from the wall. Then he realized that Chen had used his force in a clever way to lift him up along the surface of the wall as a buffer, or he would have been seriously wounded. Chen's proposal about the contest was accepted and Li became one of his disciples.

Before the competition, Chen Fake had the chance to meet with Shen San, a well-known wrestler. After exchanging compliments, Shen said candidly, "We wrestlers know little about the taijiquan you are versed in. But it seems to be a mere limbering-up exercise rather than martial art. What would you do if you had entered the contest and had to take on a wrestler by drawing the lot?"

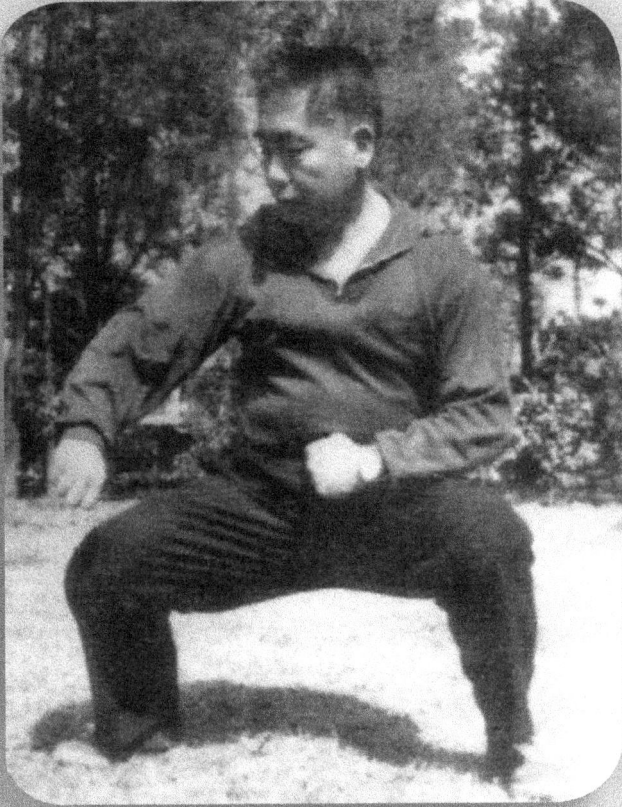

Chen Zhaokui (1928-1981), son of Chen Fake

"In real life one cannot choose an enemy when obliged to fight," Chen said. "There's always some way for one to deal with another." "How about you dealing with me?"

"Let's have a try, although I'm not so sure of myself." Chen stretched out his arms and went on, "Just hold them."

All present held their breath and were expecting a thrilling fight when the two ended it with a peal of laughter, without showing any of their combat skills.

Two days later, Shen came to Chen's training hall with some presents. "Many thanks for letting me go unharmed the other day." "The same to you," Chen replied. "It was an even score."

Chen's disciples were baffled, recalling that the two didn't fight at all. Seeing their bewilderment, the guest asked, "Didn't your master tell you everything when he came back?"

All shook their heads.

"Ah!" Shen exclaimed, giving a slap on his own leg and holding up his thumbs. "Your master is not only a wushu expert, but also a noble character. Do you think we didn't measure our strength that day? You're wrong here. As a proverb goes, 'A touch on the hand makes you understand.' I came to know I was no match for your master the moment I held his arms. He could have beaten me easily if we had not cancelled the bout by laughing it away."

After Shen San left, some of Chen's pupils asked him why he didn't knock him down, just to give him a lesson. The master turned very serious and said, "Why should I make him "lose his face" and besmirch his hard-earned reputation? Would you have me do this to you if you were in his place? Always remember: Do not do to others what you would not have them do to you."

Chen Xiao Wang

As a 19th-generation descendant of the Chen family in Chenjiagou village, where the chen-style taijiquan originated, Chen Xiaowang is now the deputy director and senior coach of the Wushu Academy of Henan Province. His grandfather Chen Fake, his father Chen Zhaoxu and his uncle Chen Zhaokui were all maestros in taijiquan. Chen Fake learnt the art from his father at eight. When he grew older, he practised the routines five times both in the morning and in the evening - a daily routine he kept up for 11 years when he helped with farm work at home.

CHEN
XIAO
WANG

19TH GENERATION DESCENDANT

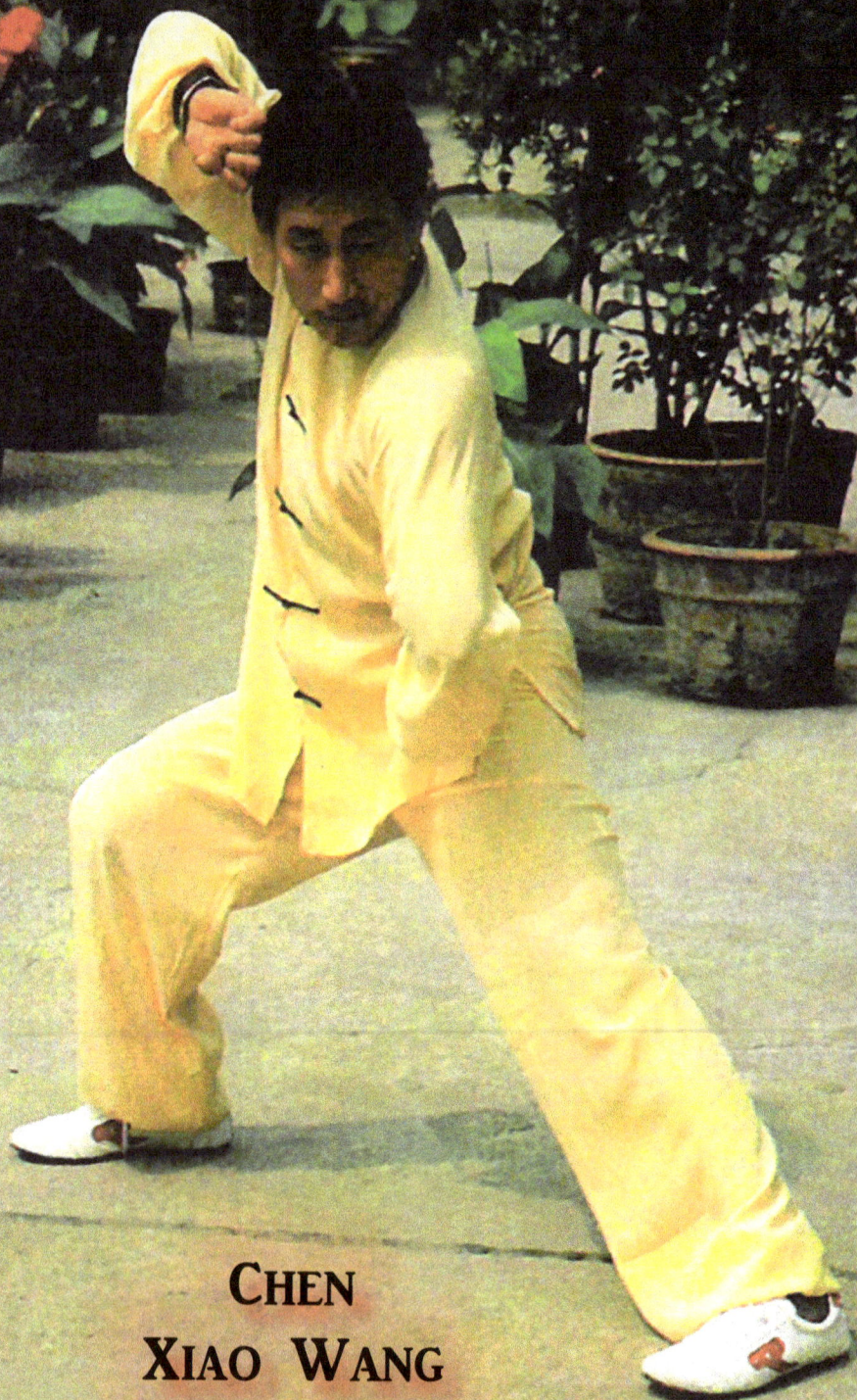

Fend off and stroke.

CHEN
XIAO WANG

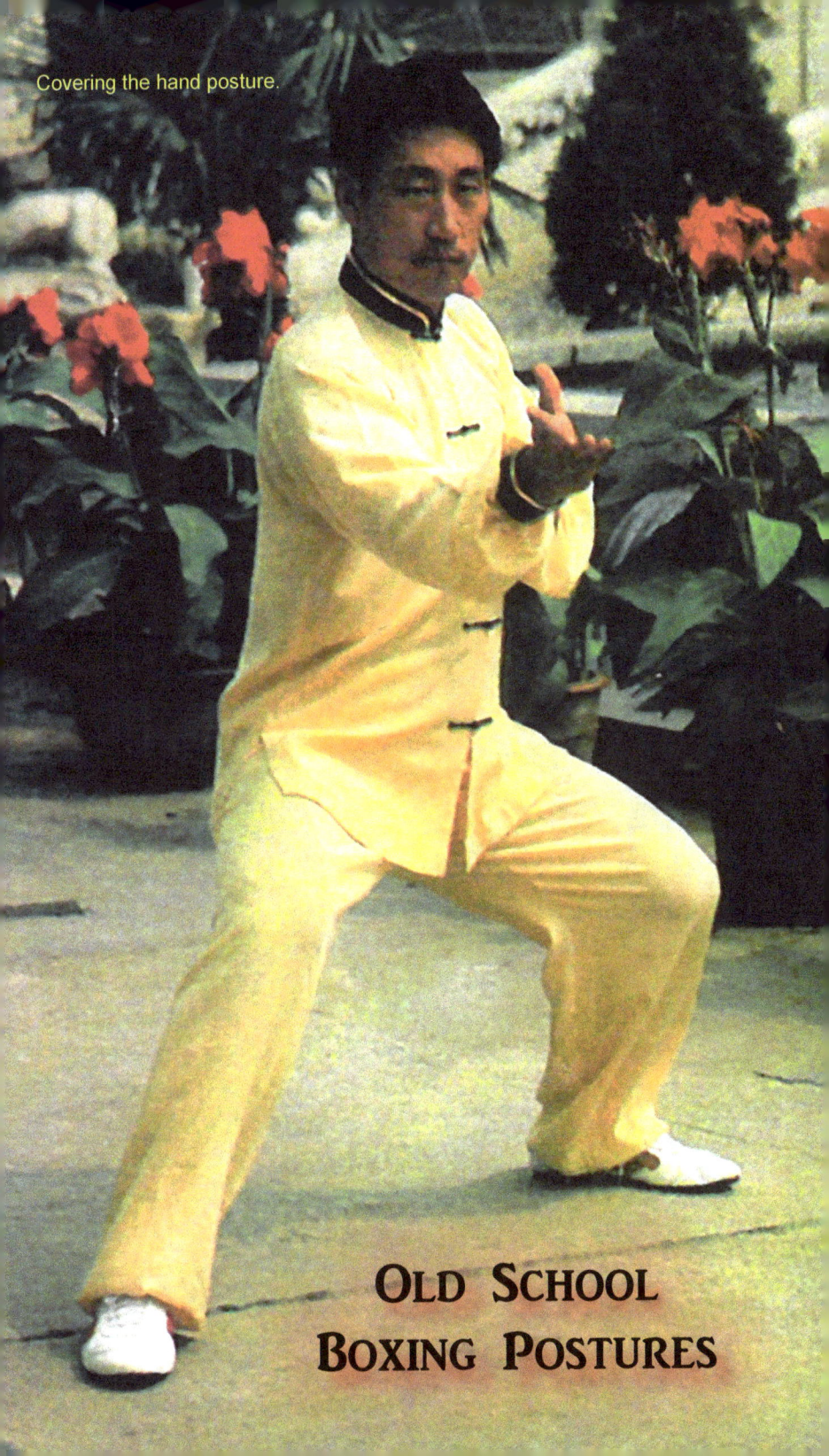

Covering the hand posture.

OLD SCHOOL
BOXING POSTURES

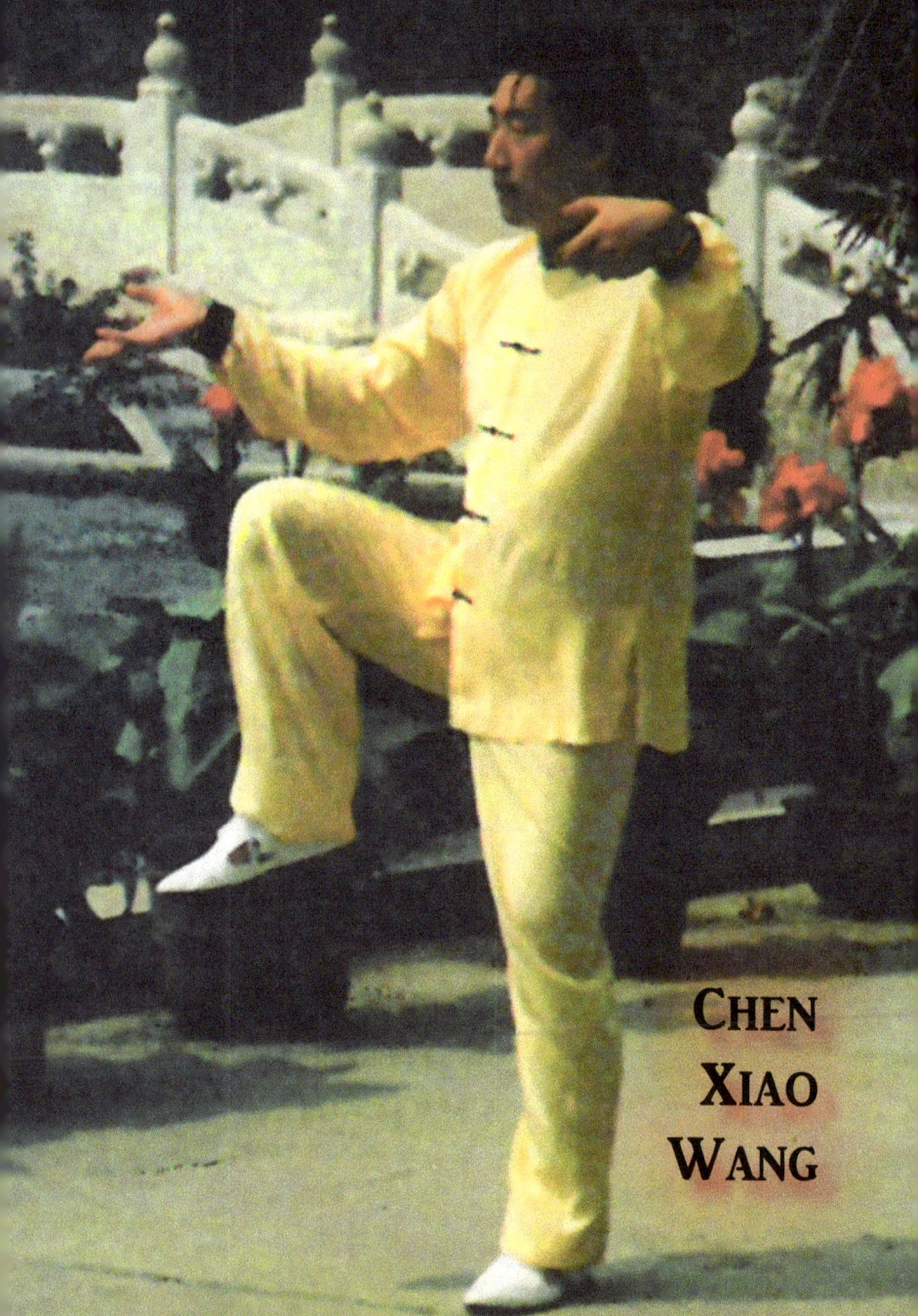

Golden Rooster stands on one leg

CHEN
XIAO
WANG

Xiaowang got a job as a purchasing agent at the General Machinery plant in the county seat of Wenxian in 1974. Though he had to travel from place to place, he persevered in practising taijiquan no matter how busy he was.

Once he was away purchasing materials for building a house for himself in his home village. He simply couldn't find any time for his daily exercises. Finally he decided to give up the plan of building his house though its walls were half completed, so that he could continue his training uninterrupted. Three years later, the walls that were left unfinished had collapsed, but his taijiquan skills had greatly improved.

He was appointed a coach at the Wushu Academy of Henan Province in 1980, what with his expertise in taijiquan and his being a direct descendant of the founder of the Chen-style. That same year he represented Henan Province at the National Wushu Tournament and won the taijiquan title. In the ensuing years, he distinguished himself as an undisputed taijiquan master by collecting more titles at national and international invitationals.

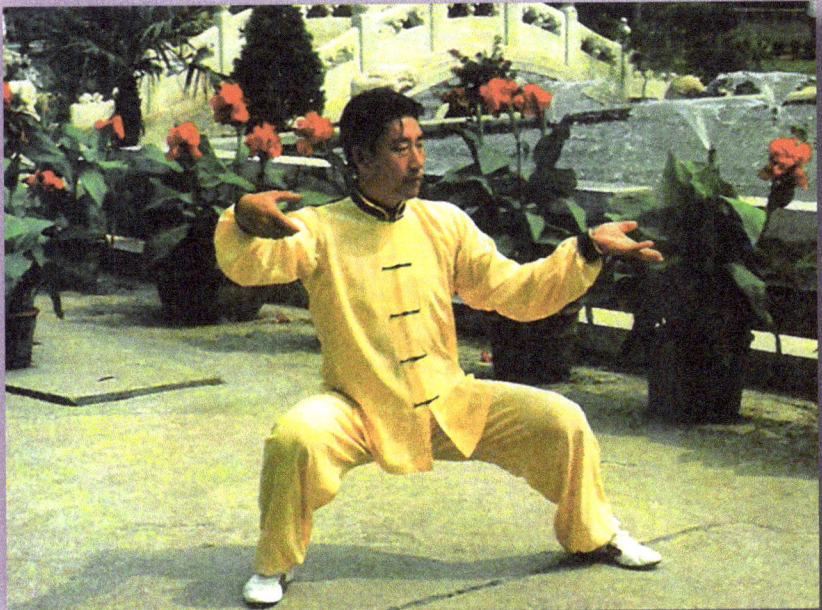

A stroke on the horse-riding stance

In March 1981 when a Japanese taijiquan group visited Henan, Chen Xiaowang defeated three Japanese masters in friendly bouts: his combat skills were highly appreciated by the guests. Recognized as a young prominent figure in the wushu community both at home and abroad, he has been invited to Japan and Singapore to pass on his skills. Moreover, quite a number of foreigners have come to Henan to learn taijiquan from him.

Chen Xiaowang has done a lot for the promotion and research of taijiquan. His simplified *Chen-style Taijiquan in 38 Forms* is regarded as a standard textbook for the beginners. From time to time he is invited to perform at exhibitions and in TV shows. The documentaries *A Visit to the Home of Taijiquan* and *Chen-Style Taijiquan*, in which he plays a major role, have been warmly received by wushu enthusiasts.

"In March 1981 when a Japanese taijiquan group visited Henan, Chen Xiaowang defeated three Japanese masters in friendly bouts: his combat skills were highly appreciated by the guests."

The Chen-style taijiquan is the oldest in China, on which all the other chief styles - Yang, Wu, Wu and Sun - are based.

Yang-style

TAIJIQUAN

Yang Luchan, Founder

(1799 - 1872)

Yang Luchan, whose original name was Yang Fukui, was born into a poor family in Nanguan Village of Yongnian County in Hebei Province. He learnt Bongquan when he was a boy and developed a pair of exceptionally strong arms.

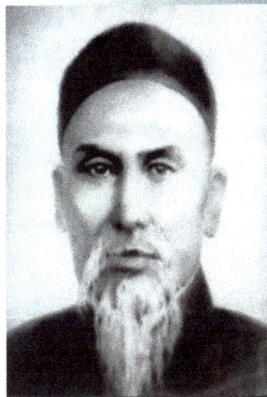

Yang Luchan

When he was old enough to work, he helped support his family by selling fine-grained yellowish soil used for making briquettes. In his late teens, he took a fancy to taijiquan and was recommended to Chen Changxing, who lived in the neighbouring Province of Henan. But it was a rule among the Chens to pass on their skills to members of the family only. Yang pretended to be mute and, through a stratagem, succeeded in staying in Chen Changxing's house where he learned taijiquan on the sly while working as a servant. Later, he became the first disciple of the Chen-style taijiquan outside the Chen family.

In 1850, Yang Luchan helped the Desheng Armed Escort Bureau to get back the large amount of silver which had been entrusted by the Prince of Duan, a member of the imperial house of the Qing Dynasty, but had been robbed by highwaymen. This won the

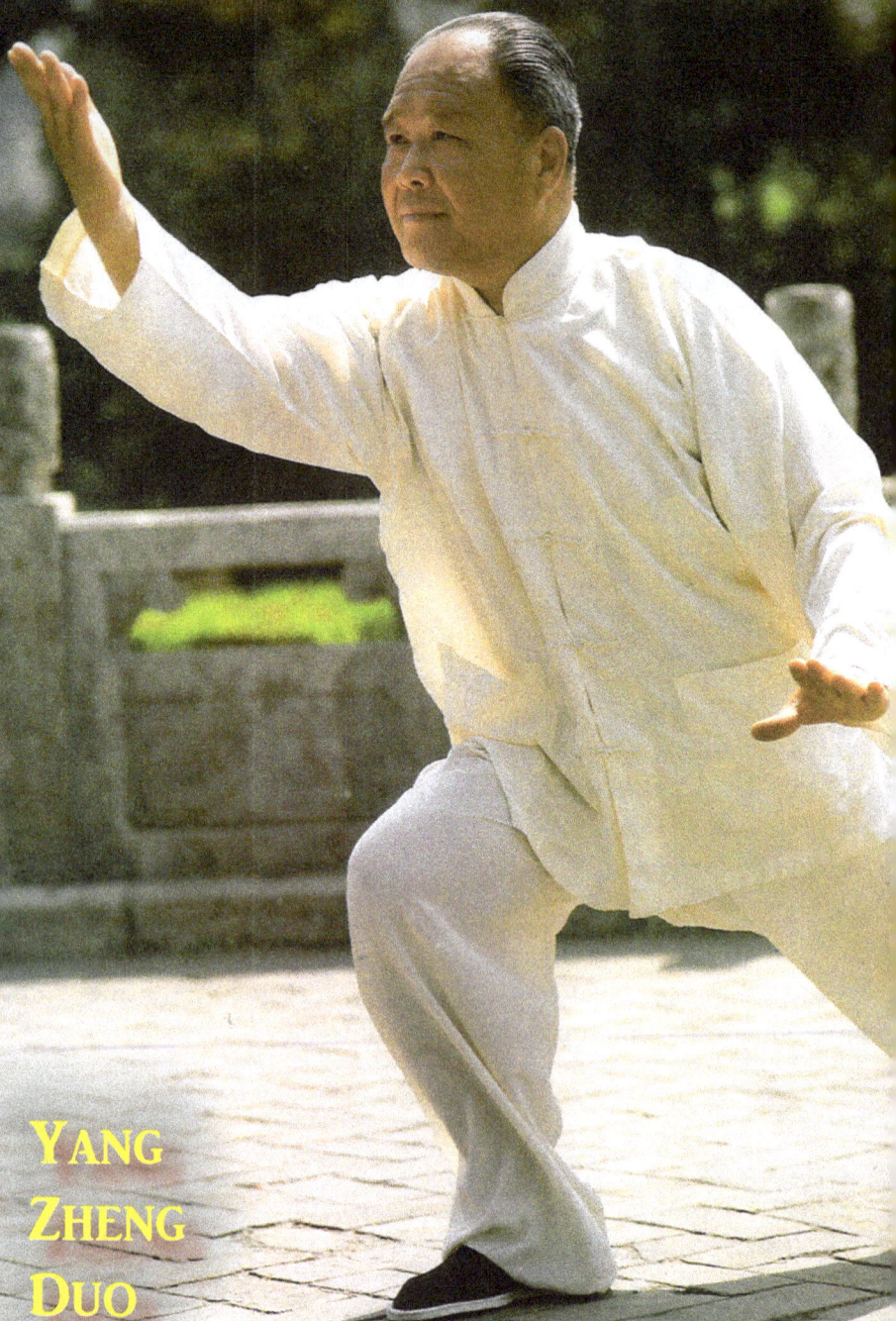

prince's favour and Yang was invited to teach wushu in his mansion. While serving under the prince, he often took time off to teach taijiquan to the common people in the city. He revised and rearranged the "old frame" of the Chen-style and created a new style of his own, which was based on a "small frame."

Further changes were made by his sons Yang Banhou and Yang Jianhou and his grandson Yang Chengfu, until it developed into the present popular Yang-style taijiquan.

Yang Luchan's disciples numbered in the hundreds. The most prominent ones included his two sons and Wu Yuxiang, Ling Shan, Wan Chun and Quan You. He had also given instruction to Wang Lanting and Li Ruidong who were in overall charge of the Prince of Duan's royal mansion. Thus, it was he who laid a solid foundation for his disciples to create more styles of taijiquan, notably Wu, Wu, Sun and Li, who made great contributions to the development of wushu by inheriting the past and opening a new epoch of taijiquan.

Yang Luchan tricks his way Into Chen's Clan

During the reign of Emperor Dao Guang (1821-1851) of the Qing Dynasty, there was a man named Yang Luchan who lived just outside the southern city gate of the county seat of Guangping (present-day Yongnian) in Hebei Province. He was very poor and made a living by selling fine-grained yellowish soil used for making briquettes. A man of sturdy build, with broad shoulders and powerful arms, he was known far and near for his great strength. His wheelbarrow was always loaded with no less than 800 catties (400 kilos) of soil, which was quite enough to meet the needs of half the inhabitants on a street. Hence his nicknames of "800 catties" and "Half the street." Toiling and moiling in this way, he could earn just enough to support his family.

On the western street in the city, there was a traditional Chinese medicine store called Tai He Tang, owned and run by people from Chenjiagou of Wenxian County in Henan Province. It was said that they were good at a kind of slow-motion shadow boxing called taijiquan and that they practised it every day with the door closed before and after opening hours. Thus no one knew exactly what it was.

One early morning Yang came to the city as usual, pushing his wheelbarrow right to the door of the store and knocked. One of the attendants let him in without any suspicion. While taking his time to unload his barrow, Yang watched the shop attendants practising tuishou (push hands) in the courtyard. Their movements were gentle and slow, as if they were swimming leisurely or feeling for fish in a river. "What kind of fighting art is this?" Yang said to himself with a sneer. Unwilling to waste his time watching such nonsense, he left right after the unloading, and thereafter he just laughed whenever people talked about taijiquan.

One day, he happened to see a crowd outside the medicine store. Hearing an exchange of angry words, he put his barrow by the roadside and edged his way through the crowd. There were the Zhao brothers from the Northern street shouting and swearing at the attendants. They wanted to return the medicine they had bought earlier and a receive a refund.

"All the medicines sold here are good," one of the attendants said. "We can return the money if you insist. But as for the medicine which is taken orally, once it is sold, we never take it back. You'll have to take your medicine away."

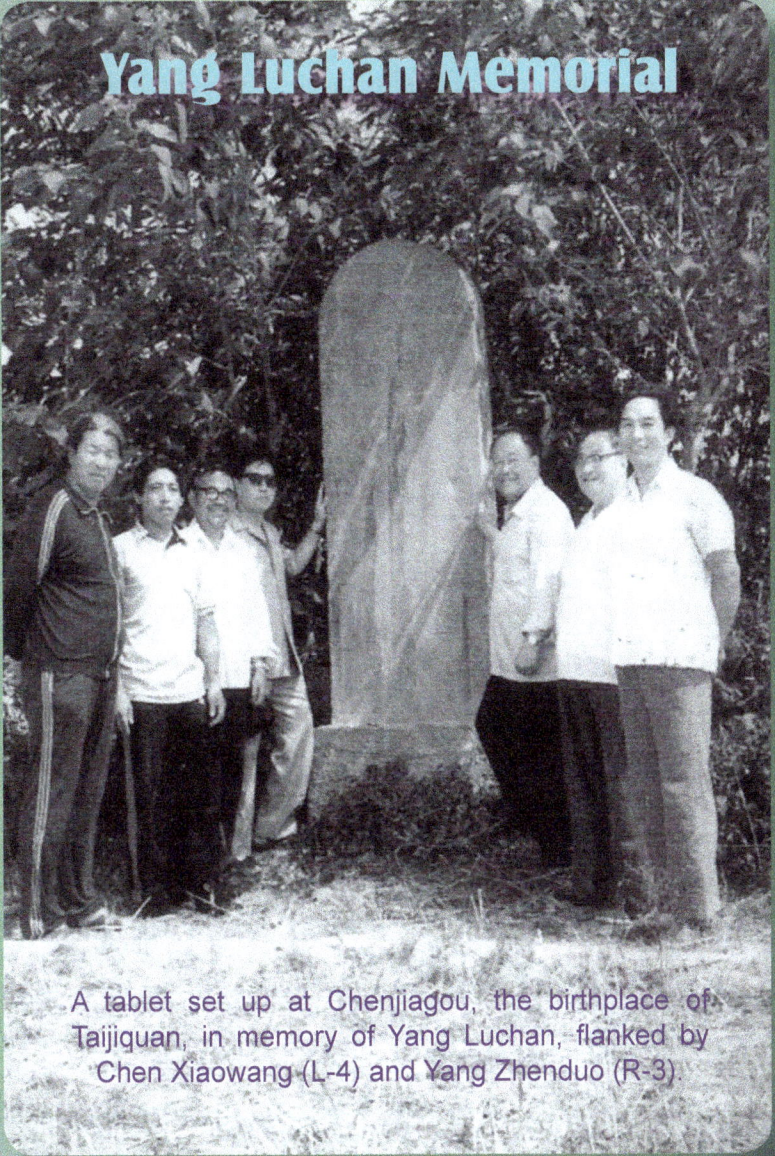

Yang Luchan Memorial

A tablet set up at Chenjiagou, the birthplace of Taijiquan, in memory of Yang Luchan, flanked by Chen Xiaowang (L-4) and Yang Zhenduo (R-3).

"We mean business today," one of the Zhaos roared. "You've got to take it back whether you like it or not!"

With this he picked up the parcel of herbal medicine and hurled it at the attendant, who caught it in his hand with amazing dexterity and, with just a flick of his wrist, threw it back, splashing the medicine all over Zhao's face. All the Zhaos rushed at the attendant.

With a seemingly effortless push, he threw them out one by one onto the street. It was only after quite a while that they were able to get to their feet. The incident created a sensation in the city. Having seen it with his own eyes, Yang Luchan was convinced of the real power of taijiquan. "It's marvelous!" he remarked. "If this young attendant is so skilful, his master must be even more terrific."

With a seemingly effortless push, he threw them out, one by one onto the street.

From then on, Yang delivered soil to the store at a regular time every day and left without collecting any money. The manager had it sent to Yang's home but it was returned intact. To find out Yang's intention, the manager invited him to a dinner on the eve of Lunar New Year's Day. After drinking had gone through three rounds, the manager asked: "There's an old saying that when someone gives you a present, he must have a request to make. If there's anything I can do for you, please let me know."

"I want to learn taijiquan."

"That's easy. But you'd better learn it from really good masters. I'll introduce you to Master Chen Changxing in Chenjiagou." Taking out a writing brush and a piece of paper, the manager immediately wrote a letter of introduction for him.

A few days later, Yang Luchan set out on his journey to Chenjiagou. It took him only four days to cover the 400 km. Chen Changxing treated him courteously to nice food and wine, but refrained from mentioning anything about taijiquan. Yang became impatient as time passed and implored Chen to accept him as a pupil.

"I've stopped practising taijiquan," Chen said, smiling. "As I've neglected it for many years, I'm afraid I may waste your time. You'd better learn from someone else."

Yang's heart sank when he heard Chen's words which amounted to a flat refusal. No matter how he pleaded, Chen was adamant. Yang had no choice but to bow out.

It was in the depth of winter. Snow began to fall in big flakes one late afternoon and did not stop until the next morning. When the attendants in Chen Changxing's house opened the door to sweep away the snow by the roadside, they saw someone lying on the ground. It was a beggar in tatters with a dirty, dark face. He was shivering with cold and seemed to have lost consciousness. They ran into the house and reported it to Chen Changxing, who came out and told his men to carry the beggar inside. When the poor man finally came to, they found he could not utter a word. He was a mute! Feeling sorry for the beggar, Chen Changxing let him stay. Being physically strong, the beggar did all kinds of work, carrying buckets of water from a nearby well, sweeping the floor and cleaning the house, making fire and cooking. His diligence and thoroughness won the heart of everyone. The beggar was none other than Yang Luchan.

Having successfully concealed his identity, Yang Luchan did household chores in the daytime, and in the evening when the family and Chen's disciples started practising taijiquan, he would stand close by and watch attentively, memorizing every movement. On the fifteenth day of every lunar month when there was a full moon, the Chen family held a contest at night, which was a special attraction to Yang. Since he was a mute, the Chens did not mind his presence.

Every night when the whole family had gone to sleep, Yang would get up and practise all the parts he had memorized. Three years passed without incident. Then one night as Yang was practising as usual, Chen Changxing happened to get up. When he saw someone doing taiji exercises in the courtyard, he called out, "Who's there?"

"It's me, Luchan," Yang blurted out in his unguarded moment.

Chen Changxing asked in great surprise: "You're a mute. How can you speak now?"

"I'm Yang Luchan," Yang said in an apologetic voice as he kowtowed. "I came to you three years ago from Guangping with a letter of introduction to learn taijiquan." Then he told how he had disguised himself as a dumb beggar to get himself accepted and how he had learnt taijiquan by watching and practising it late at night for three years.

Deeply moved by Yang's determination, Chen asked him to show how much he had learnt. Taking off his jacket, Yang demonstrated all the routines he had picked up. His performance, skillful and true to the Chen-style, compared favorably with that of Chen Changxing's children and nephews.

"Since you've been working so hard at it," Chen said, "you may stay here for another three years. I'll teach you personally."

Yang was overjoyed and kowtowed again and again. From then on, the two got along so well that they looked like father and son. Chen passed on to his new disciple all the essentials of taijiquan and combat skills with bare hands or weapons and the ways of training inner strength. When he finally took his leave and returned to his hometown, Yang was a proficient and versatile wushu master.

Yang Chengfu

(1883 - 1936)

The Man Who Set the Pattern

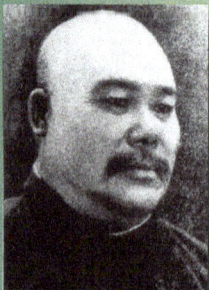

Yang Chengfu, alias Yang Caoqing, was born in Yongnian County, Hebei Province, as a grandson to Yang Luchan, founder of the Yang-style taijiquan, and the third son of Yang Jianhou. It was he who finalized this style into the present-day form that is popular both at home and abroad.

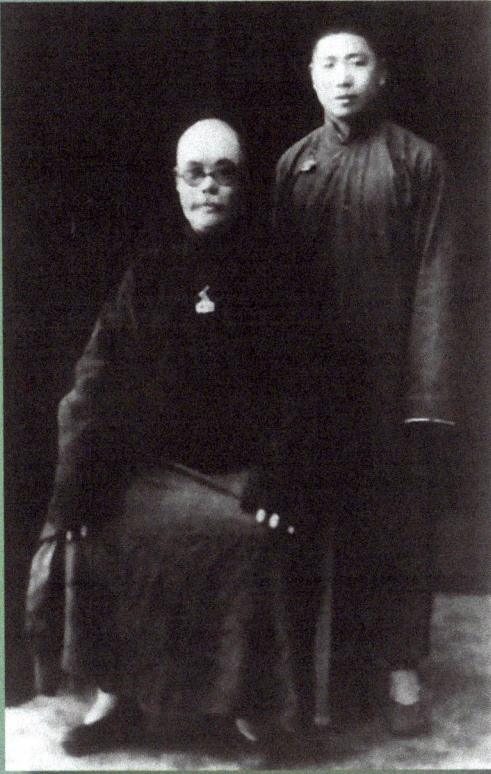

Yang Chengfu and his pupil, a young Fu
Zhongwen, in Guangzhou, 1932

Learning taijiquan from his father since early childhood, Yang Chengfu showed great talent and was quick to get the hang of it, especially the "middle frame" of Yang-style passed on by his grandfather to his father and uncle Yang Banhou, both of whom had taught wushu in the Prince of Duan's mansion and enjoyed a great reputation in Beijing.

As a grown-up, Yang Chengfu was invited by the Beijing Sports Society to coach wushu in the city and then went to Wuhan, Nanjing, Guanzhou, Shanghai and Hangzhou to teach the Yang-style taijiquan.

Because of his simplicity, modesty, gentleness and eagerness for perfection, which he seemed to have inherited from his grandfather, Yang Chengfu was loved by all his disciples, who were scattered all over the country. During his stay in Wuhan, he accepted a challenge by a local wushu master versed in swordsmanship. Wielding a mere makeshift sword of bamboo, Yang defeated his opponent who was armed with a real sword of steel. He apologized profusely for having hurt his opponent's wrist unintentionally during the fight.

While in Hong Kong, Yang was pitted against a well-known master of the southern school, who pounced on him like a hungry tiger but was thrown several metres away - with a mere jerk of Yang's forefinger! In Hangzhou, where he acted as the dean of Zhejiang Province Wushu Academy, Yang created another sensation among the wushu circles by overcoming an insolent challenger, this time with a short cudgel against a long spear.

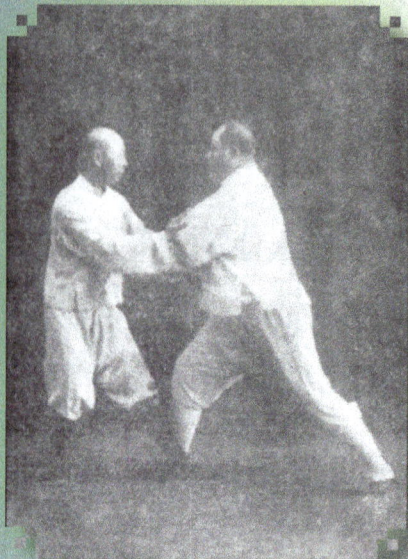

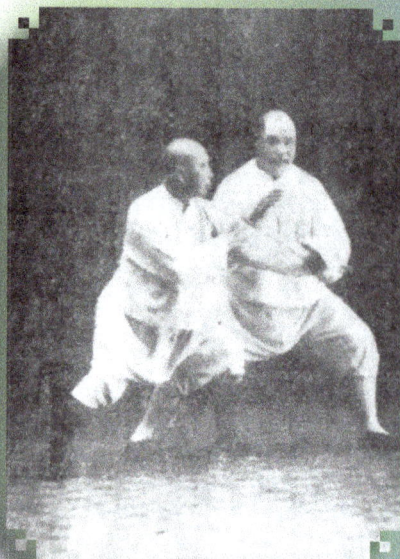

Yang Chengfu in paired training: tuishou pushing hands

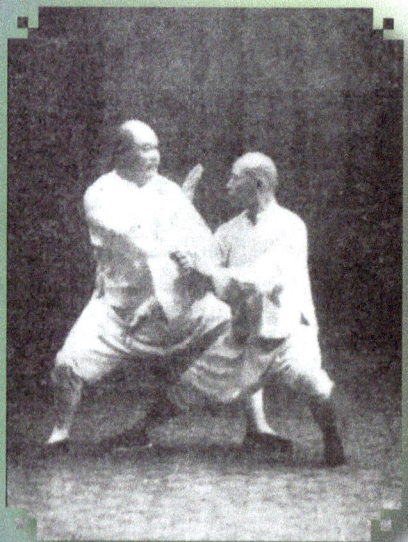

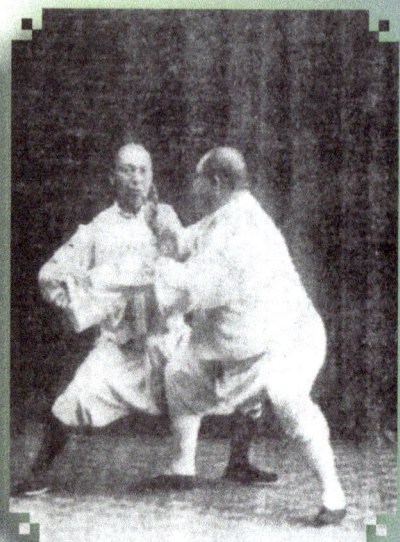

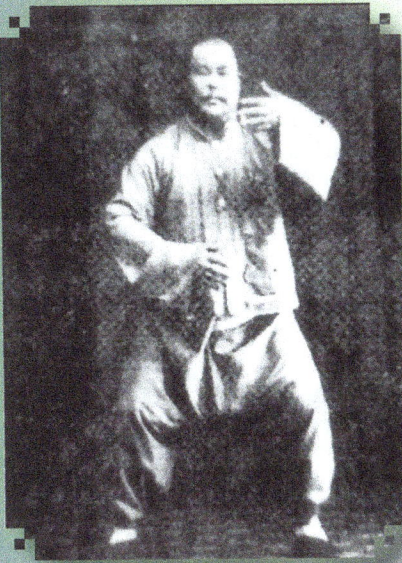

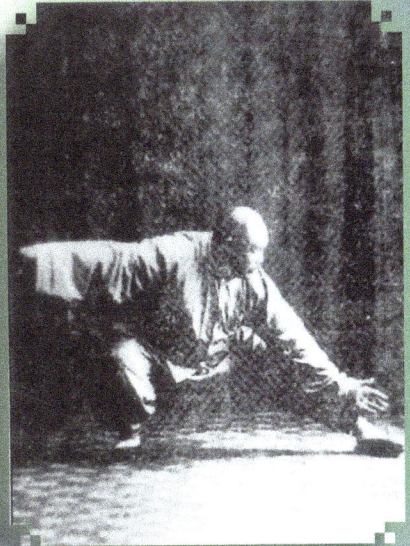

Yang Chengfu in solo training: shadowboxing postures

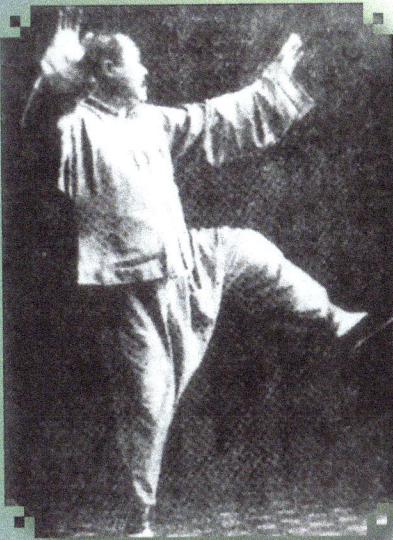

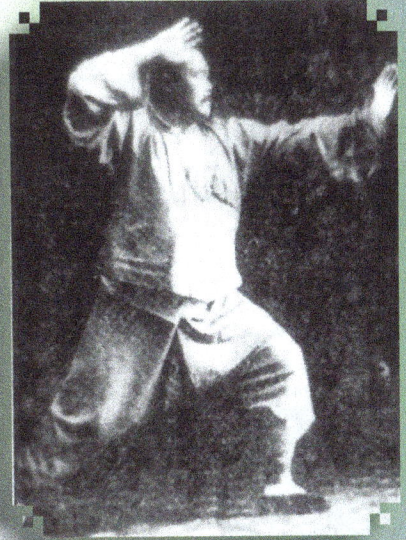

The Yang-style taijiquan was initiated by Yang Luchan and revised by Yang Banhou in its frame, or amplitude of the movements, but it was Yang Chengfu who brought it to perfection and the pinnacle of fame by imbuing into the whole set elements of grace, fluency, suppleness, close-knit composition and a combination of softness and hardness – a set of exercises that is easy to learn for the beginners.

In 1925, Yang Chengfu asked one of his disciples, Chen Weiming, to write a book entitled "Taijiquan," with detailed captions to Yang's

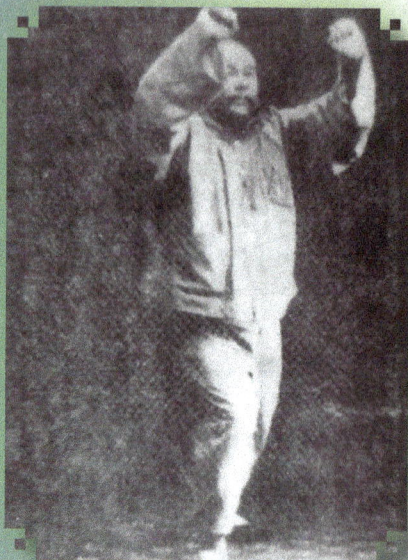

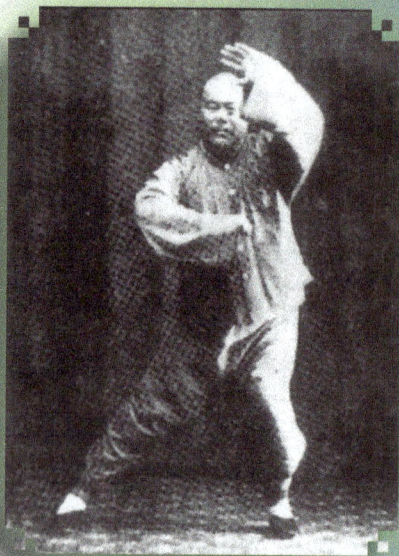

Yang Chengfu in solo training: shadowboxing postures

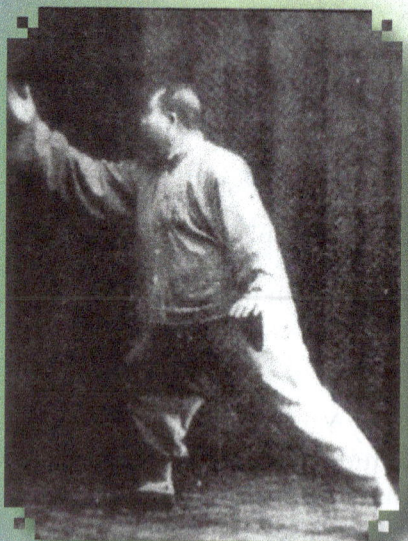

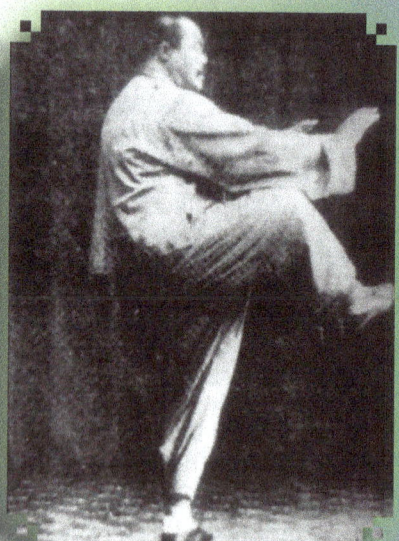

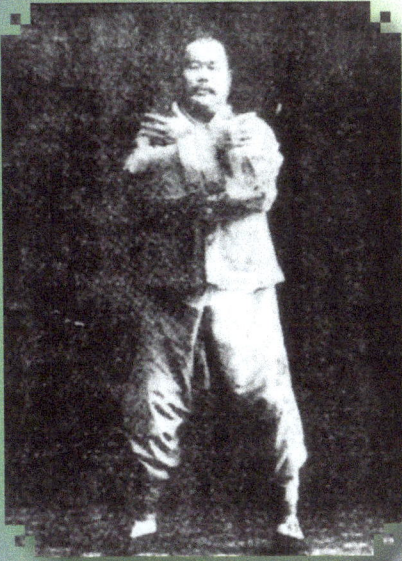

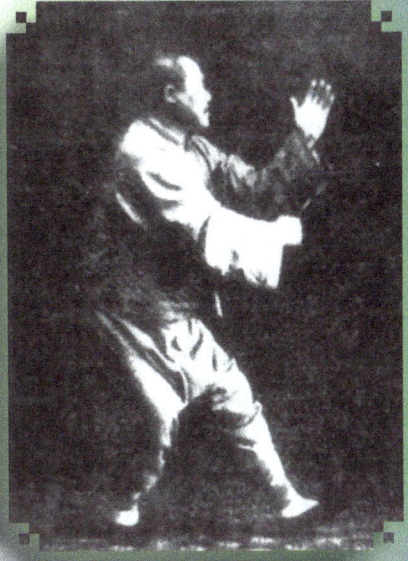

Yang Chengfu in solo training: shadowboxing postures

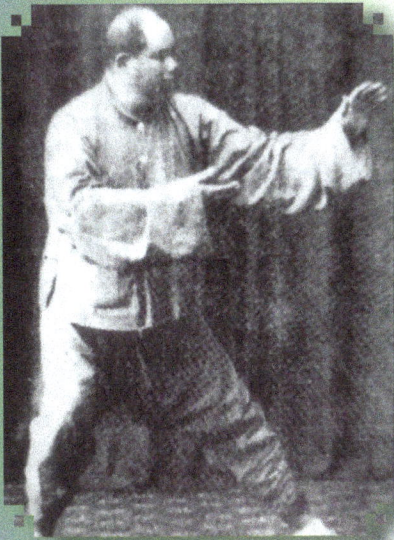

pictures as illustrations. In 1931, Yang had all the pictures retaken and compiled into *The Methods of Taijiquan*, which was revised two years later into *A Complete Book of Taijiquan*. These works are now regarded as classics on the Yang-style taijiquan, and have provided the basis for all the taijiquan routines in 24, 88 and 48 forms compiled and promulgated by the State Physical Culture and Sports Commission of the People's Republic of China since the '50s. This fact explains why Yang Chengfu has been universally acclaimed as a most important personage in China's taijiquan movement.

As director of the Wudang School under the Central Wushu Academy in Nanjing, Yang Chengfu had a large following throughout the country, of whom mention may be made of such celebrities as Chen Yuebo, Yan Zhongkui, Cui Yishi, Wang Shendong, Niu Chunming, Li Chunnian, Chen Weiming, Wu Jiangchuan, Tian Zhaolin, Dong Yingjie, Zhu Guiting and Zheng Manqing, as well as his four sons, viz., Yang Zhenming, Yang Zhenji, Yang Zhenguo and Yang Zhenduo.

Yang Zhenduo

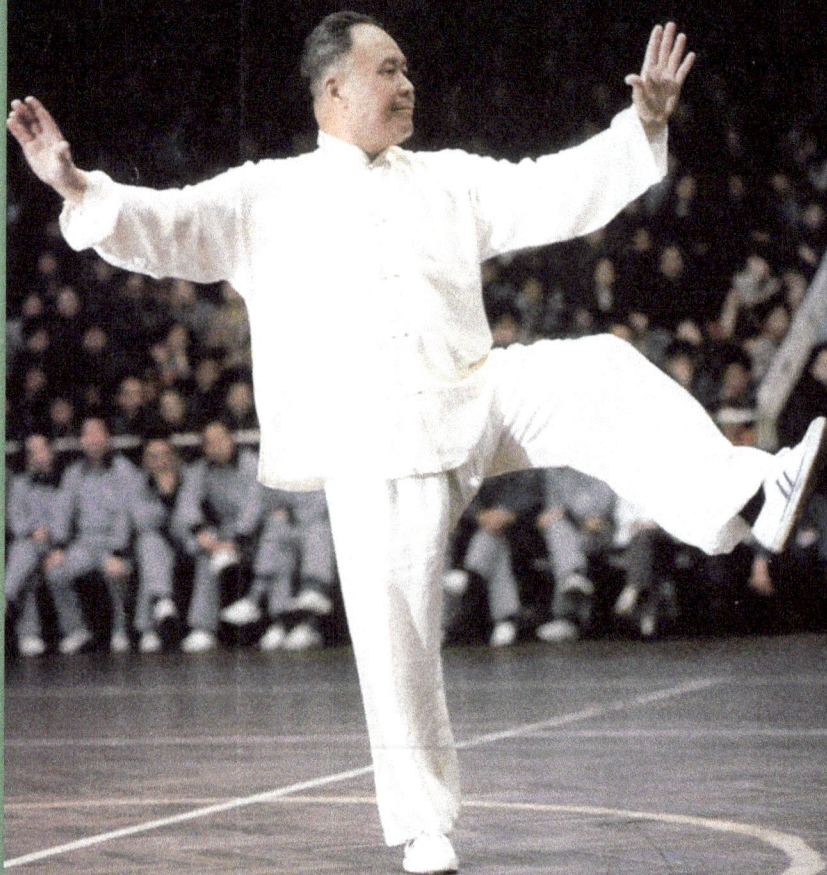

Fourth Generation Inheritor

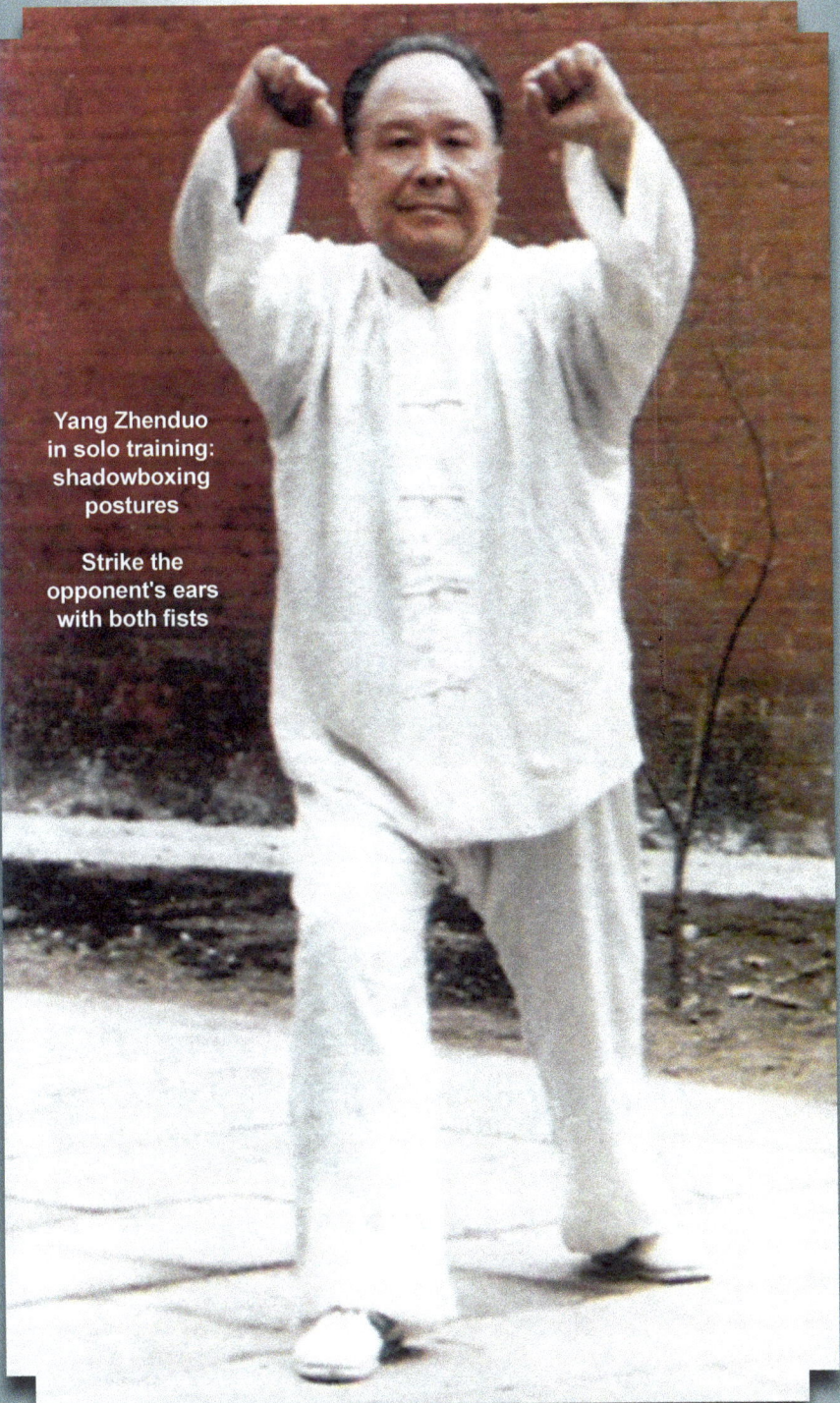

Yang Zhenduo
in solo training:
shadowboxing
postures

Strike the
opponent's ears
with both fists

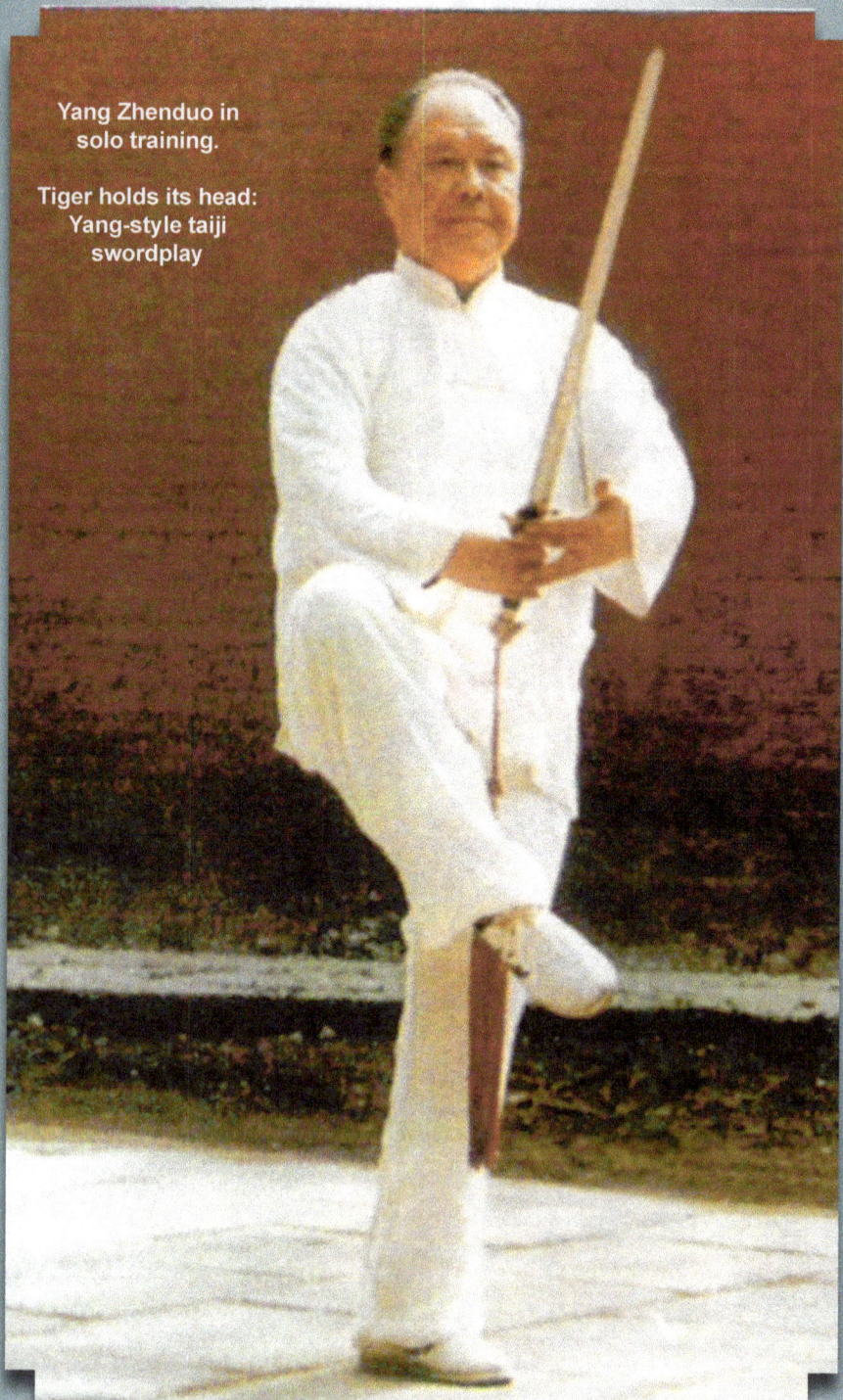

Yang Zhenduo in
solo training.

Tiger holds its head:
Yang-style taiji
swordplay

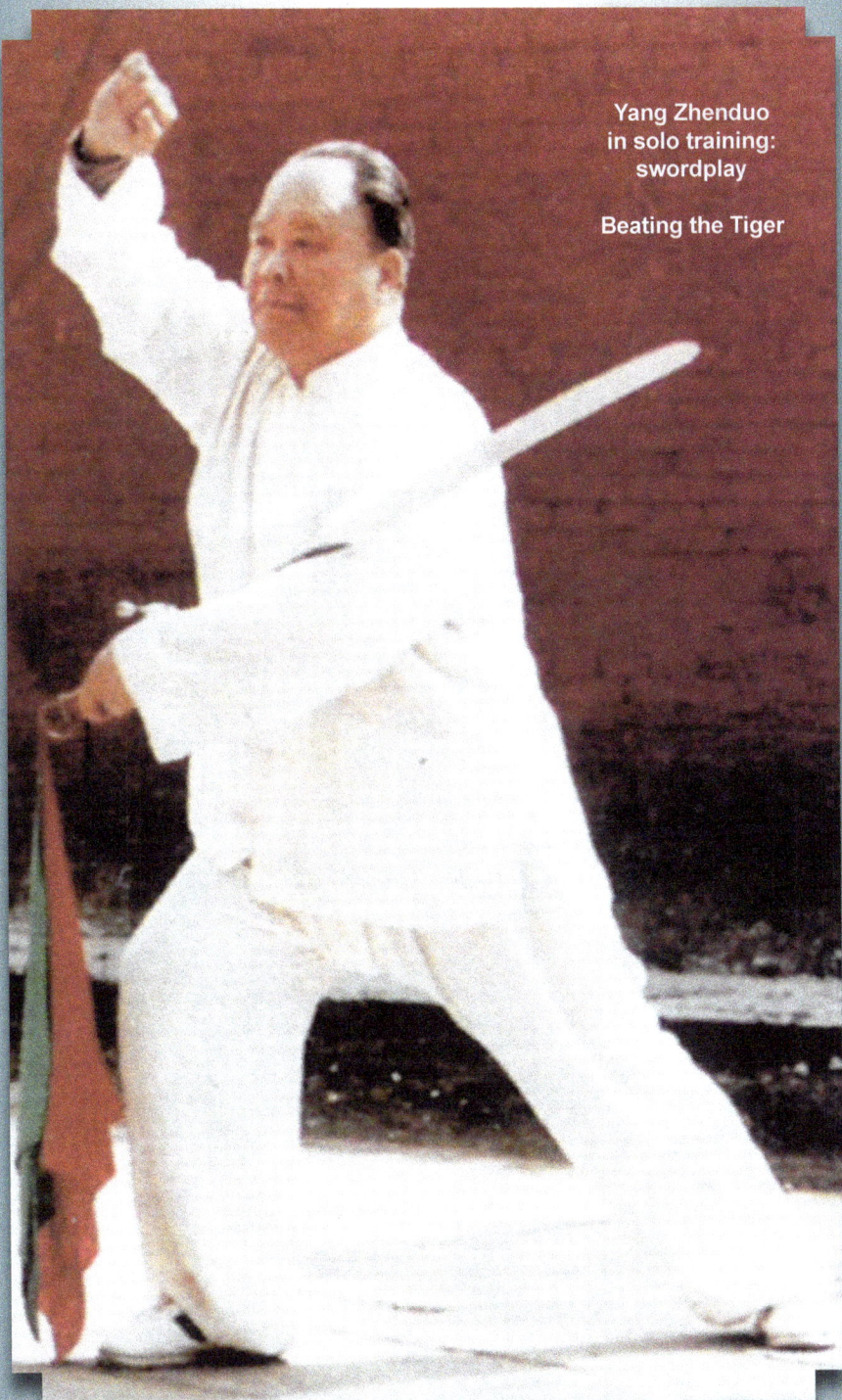

Yang Zhenduo
in solo training:
swordplay

Beating the Tiger

Yang Zhenduo
in solo training;
shadowboxing
postures

Brush the knee and
step on the left

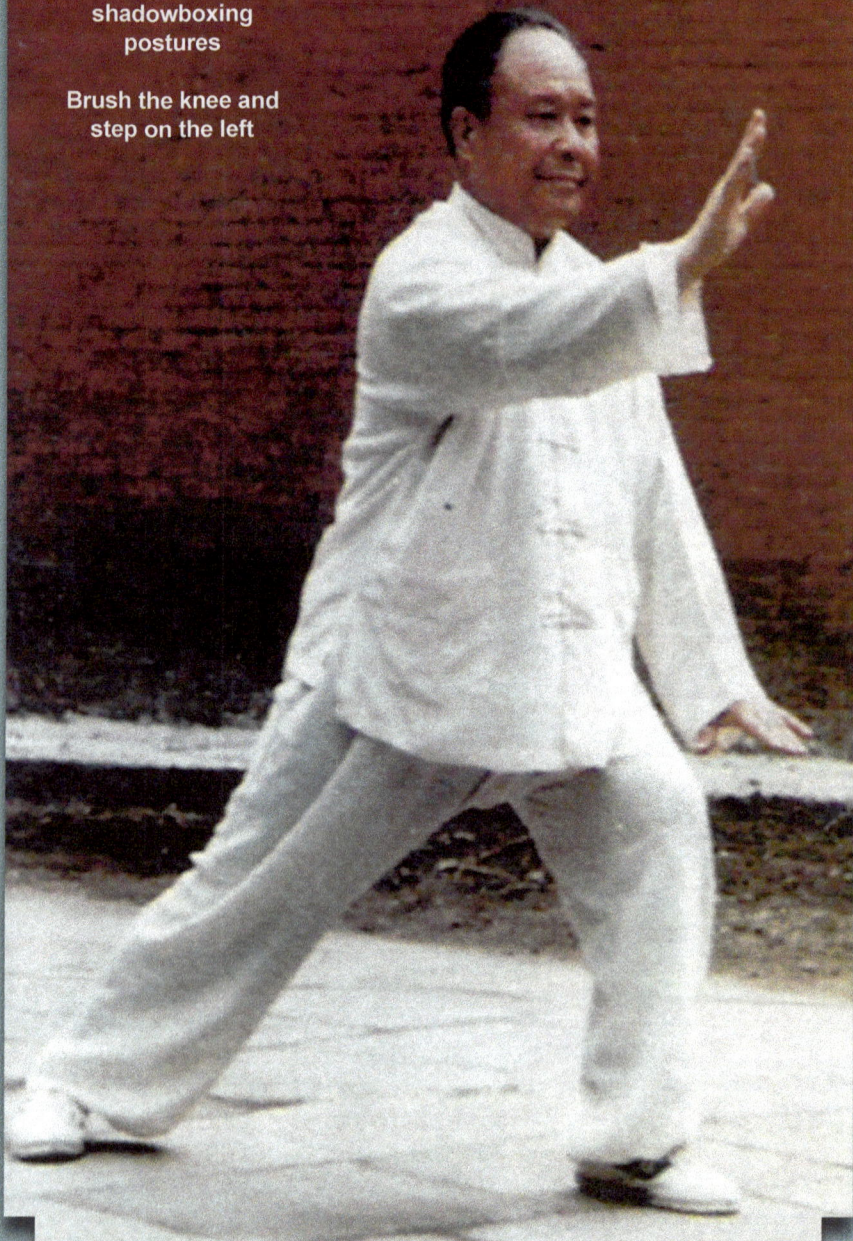

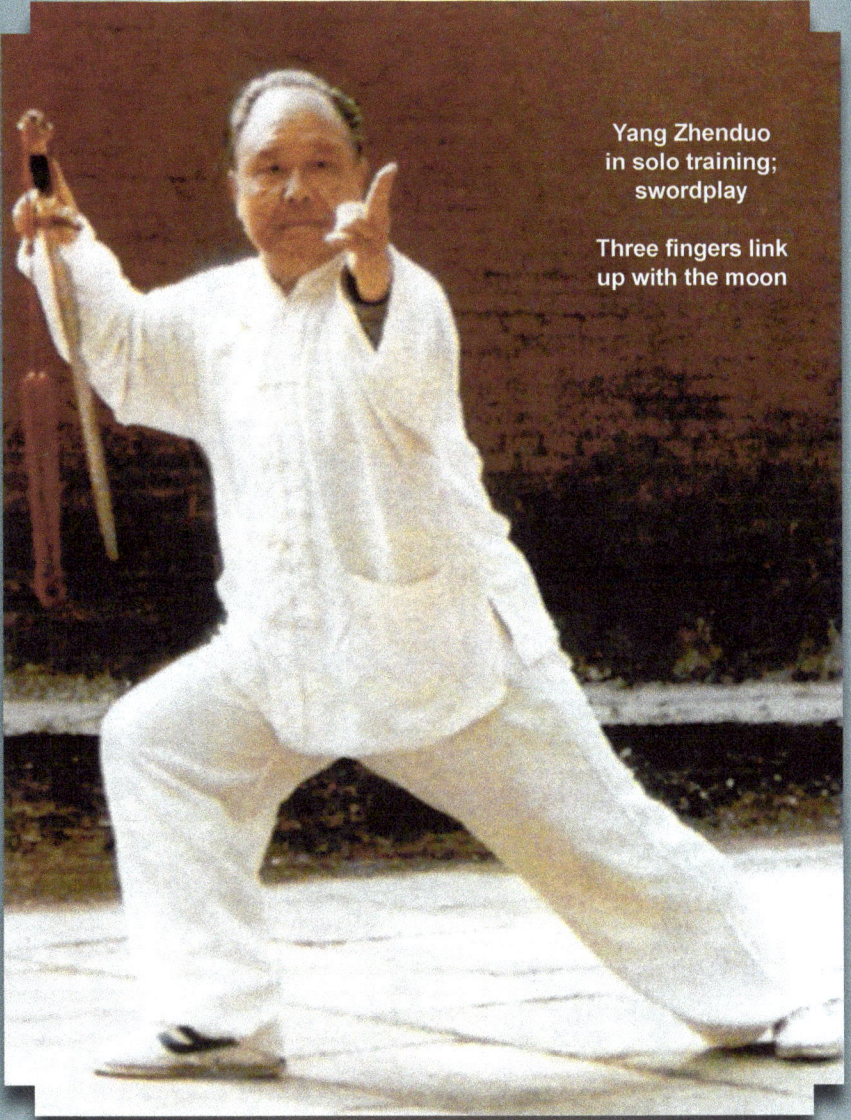

Yang Zhenduo
in solo training;
swordplay

Three fingers link
up with the moon

Yang Zhenduo

Fourth generation Inheritor

Born in 1926, in Yongnian County, Hebei Province, Yang Zhenduo is the great grandson of Yang Luchan, founder of the Yang-style taijiquan. He started learning this important school under his father

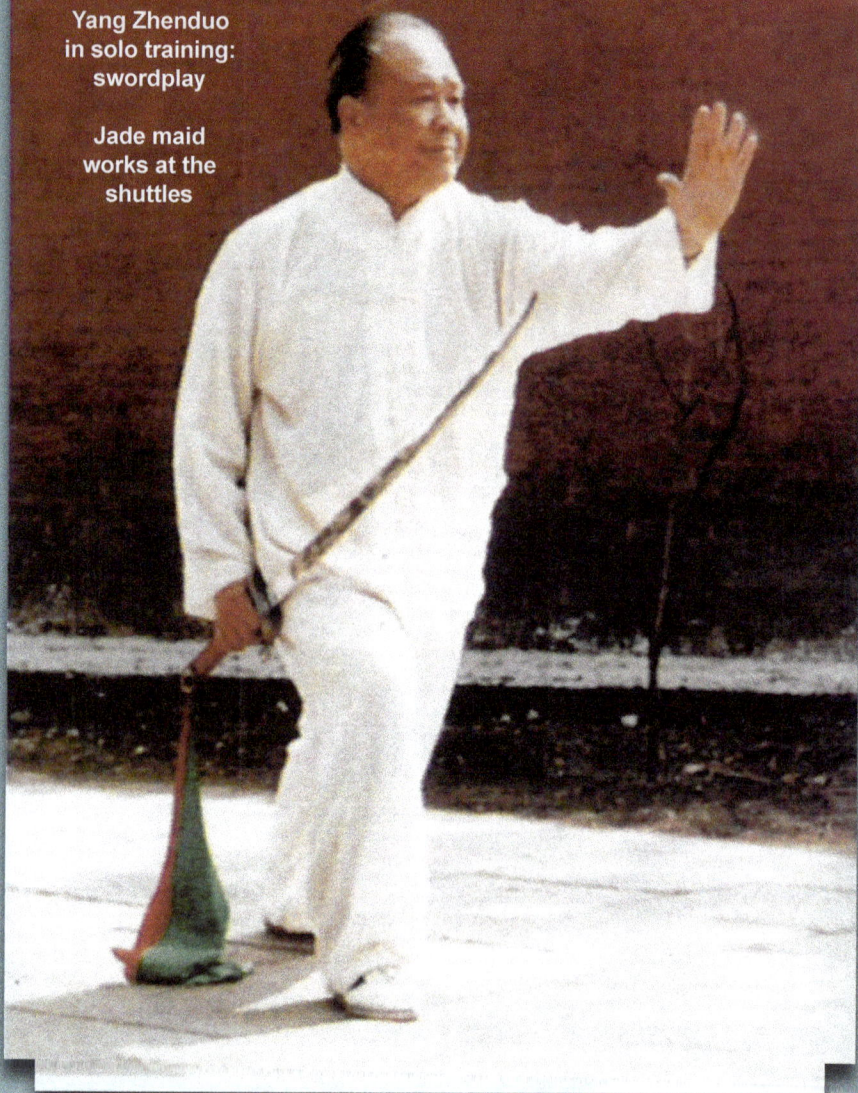

Yang Zhenduo in solo training: swordplay

Jade maid works at the shuttles

Yang Chengfu. For more than half a century, he has practiced it every day, sometimes repeating a movement thousands of times at a stretch, until he was so exhausted that he could hardly stand on his feet. It was thus that he attained perfection for the whole set of exercises on his father's pattern and style.

In 1961, he was invited to demonstrate at the Sports Palace in Shanghai, in the presence of many enthusiasts who tried to compare his performance with the illustrations in a book on his father's routine. Everything looked exactly the same - without the slightest departure from the orthodox Yang-style.

More and more people came from the neighboring cities, including Wuxi, Changshu and Hangzhou, to watch Yang Zhenduo's demonstrations.

Then he came to Shanxi Province, where he has taught more than 10,000 followers during the past three decades. He was elected President of the Yang-style Taijiquan Association in 1982 when it was founded in Shanxi.

In the following three years, he was invited to demonstrate at national wushu or taijiquan meetings in Shanghai, Guangzhou and Nanjing and won the honorable title of "Renowned Taijiquan Master" at an international contest of taiji boxing and swordplay held in Wuhan, Hebei. In addition, he was elected Honorary President of the French Taiji Association.

In 1985, together with his colleagues Li Tianji and Li Binquan, he attended a taijiquan exhibition in Singapore, where he was warmly applauded by the audience and press for his sterling performances as an epitome of what is best in taijiquan with its flowing, graceful, light and continuous movements and a combination of hardness and softness.

Then the three masters opened a three month clinic in Singapore, with Yang Zhenduo held in esteem as the fourth-generation inheritor of the genuine Yang-style taijiquan. In the next two years, Yang was invited to France twice, where he taught more than 300 people of 16 different nationalities. In recent years, he has received one batch after another of taijiquan enthusiasts from Singapore, Japan, France, Germany, USA, and Australia. Though retired in 1985, he has been working untiringly for an intensive study and broad spread of the Yang-style taijiquan, as part of a worldwide effort to internationalize wushu for the benefit of mankind. Thinking that only the first step has been taken, Yang has dedicated his whole life to this noble cause.

Yang Sidelight

The founder of this style was Yang Luchan (1799-1872). Born into a poor family in Yongnian County, Hebei Province, he worked as a servant in Chenjiagou in Henan Province, where he had the opportunity to learn martial arts from his master Chen Changxing. Then he returned to his homeland where he became an instructor of the Chen-style taijiquan. Knowing how to avoid and subdue forceful blows in fighting, Yang Luchan gained a reputation for his "cotton boxing," also known as "tender boxing" or "softening boxing." Later he went to Beijing and taught many nobles in the Qing court. Because of his superb fighting art, some people called him "Yang the Invincible," a title to be inherited by his first son Yang Banhou (1837-1892).

To adapt taijiquan exercises to his disciples, Yang Luchan omitted the most difficult movements that involved explosive force, such as forward leaps and foot stamping. It underwent further revisions by his third son Yang Jianhou (1839-1917) and grandson Yang Chengfu (1883-1936), until it was fixed into the "big frame" of the Yang-style, which enjoys the greatest popularity today. After 1928, Yang Chengfu travelled widely and spread his unique style to many cities, including Nanjing, Shanghai, Zhenjiang, Hangzhou, Guangzhou and Wuhan.

The Yang-style taijiquan is characterized by simplicity, fluidity, natural grace and a combination of softness and hardness. It may be performed in a high, middle or low body position, to be chosen by the practitioner according to his age, sex and fitness level.

This precious picture was taken at the ancient Qi Xia Temple, located to the northeast of Nanking, in 1982. They are the renowned inheritors of taijiquan. At the time, (L-R) Yang Zhenduo (Yang) was 57; Ma Yueliang (Wu) was 82; Wu Yinghua (Wu) 78; Sun Jianyuan (Sun); Chen Xiaowang 36; and Shi Meiling (Wu Yinghua's pupil). Scattering everywhere they have popularized taiji for the health of the people!

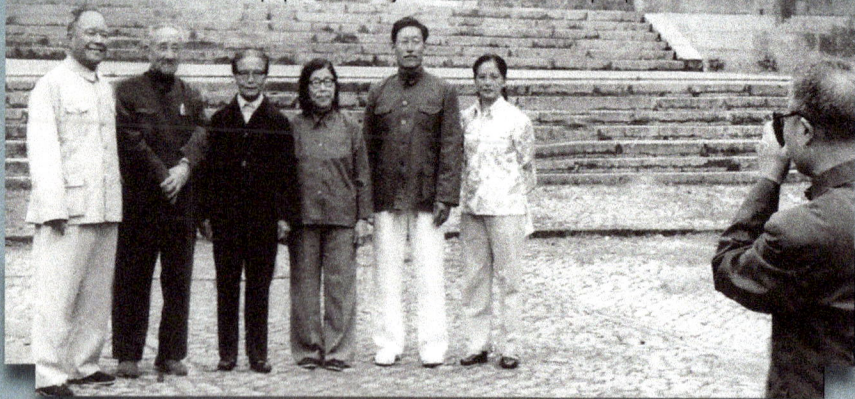

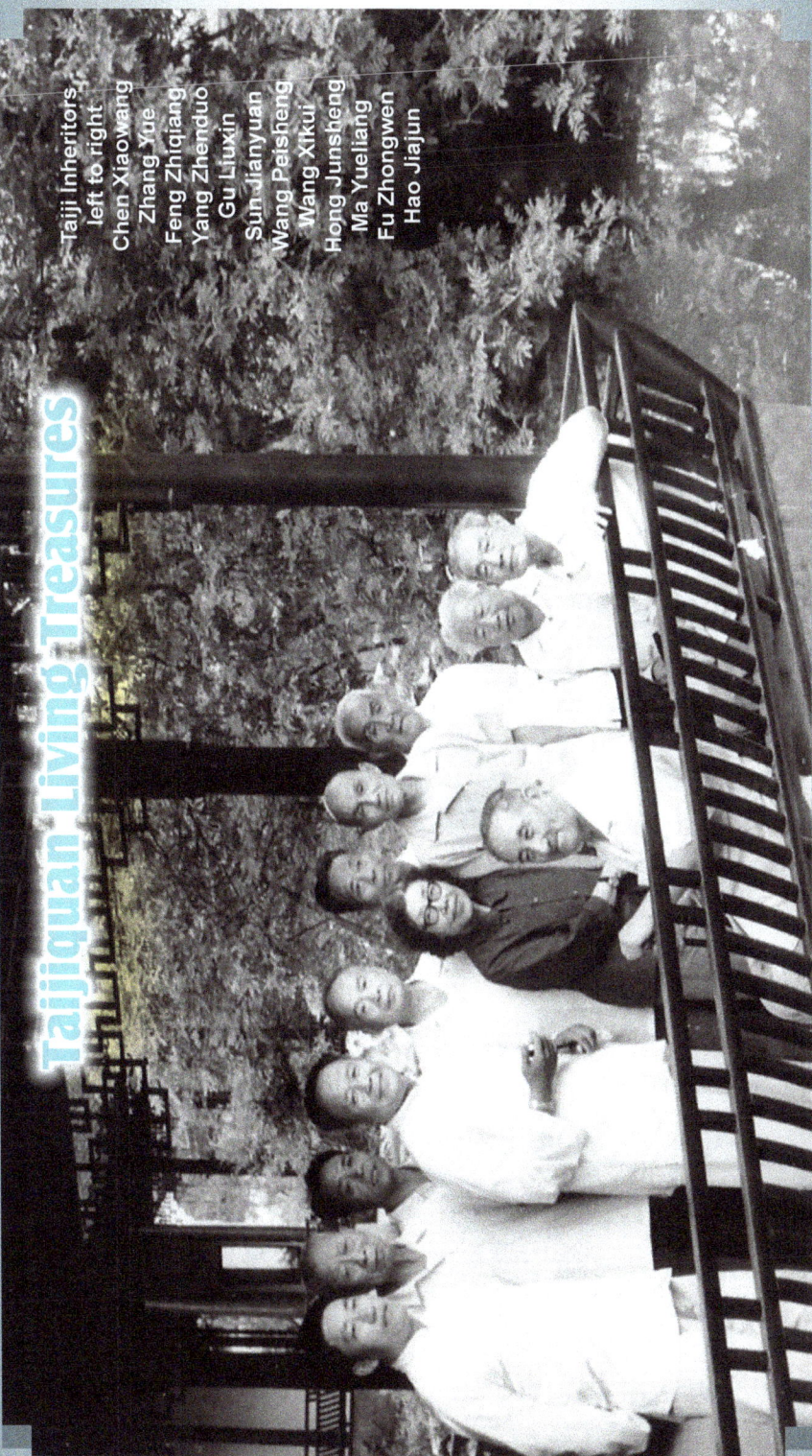

Taijiquan Living Treasures

Taiji Inheritors:
left to right
Chen Xiaowang
Zhang Yue
Feng Zhiqiang
Yang Zhenduo
Gu Liuxin
Sun Jianyuan
Wang Peisheng
Wang Xikui
Hong Junsheng
Ma Yueliang
Fu Zhongwen
Hao Jiajun

PLUM FLOWER
PEG SOCIETY

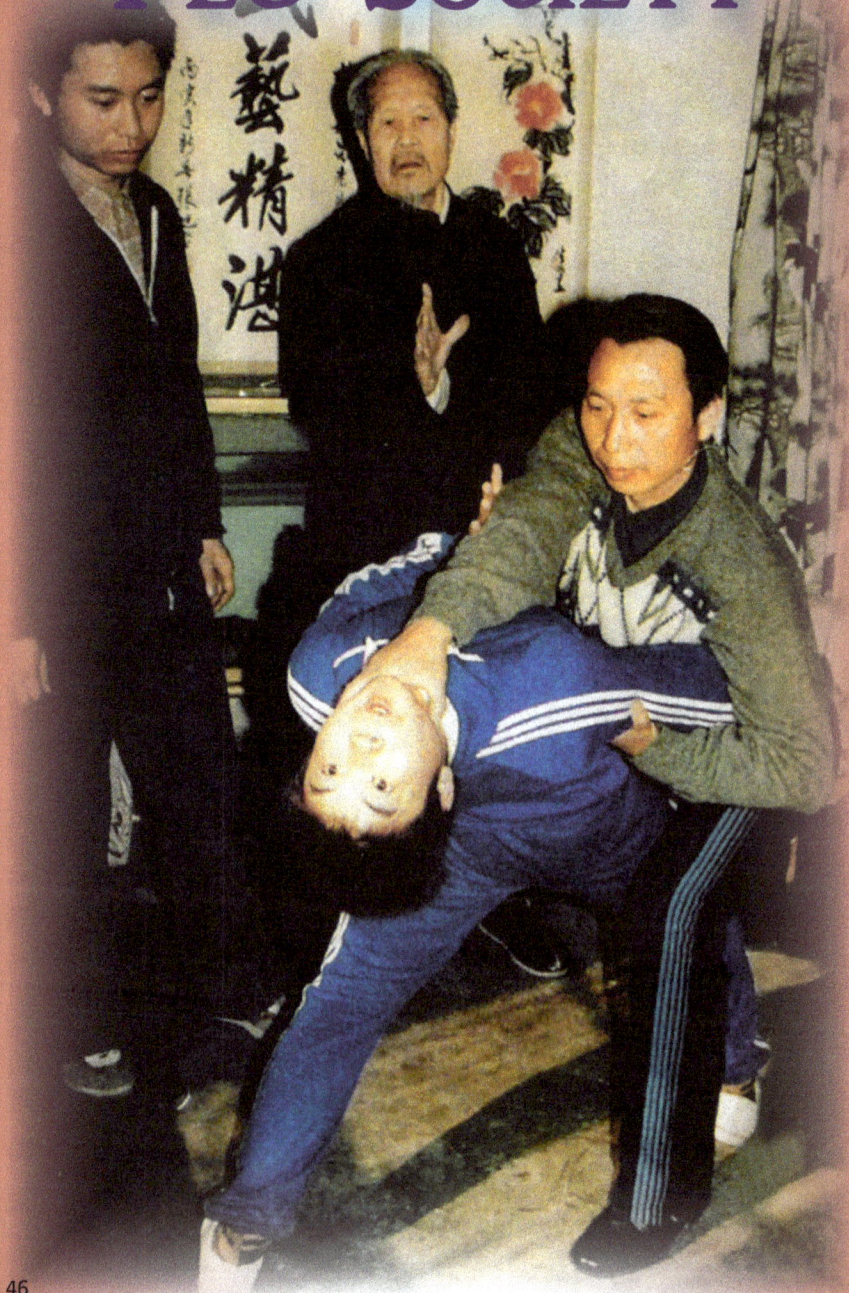

Plum Flower in Bloom

Han Qichang, alias Han Shijie, was born in Yuantou Village, Shenxian County, Hebei Province. He apprenticed himself at age 12 to two retired bodyguards, Wang Yudong and Han Yuting, who were versed in kicking skills, and three years later to Li Cunyi who was well known for his form-and-will exercises and nicknamed "Broadsword Li" for his unrivaled proficiency with this weapon. Li was involved in the Yihetuan

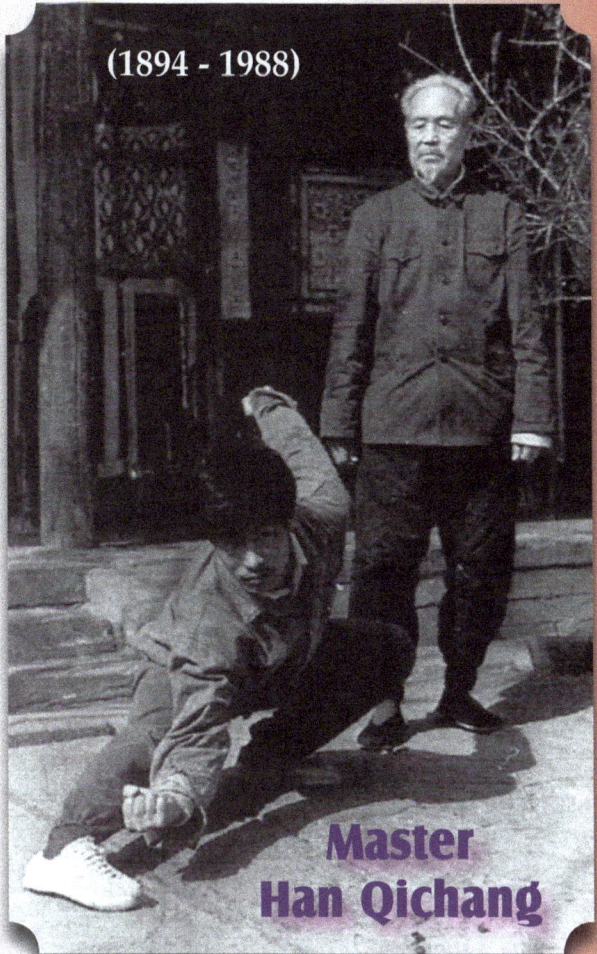

(1894 - 1988)

Master Han Qichang

Above: Han giving tips to a practitioner. Opposite: Han coaching his son Han Jianzhong (R-1)

Movement, an anti-imperialist armed struggle waged by north China peasants and handicraftsmen at the turn of this century. Han would steal out of his house at midnight to get lessons from Broadsword Li, who thought highly of Han's diligence, talent and honesty and passed on all his knowledge to him without reservation.

Eager to learn more wushu schools, Han approached another master, Li Guisui, who taught him everything he knew about the martial art with hooks.

Han had unusual muscular strength. One day he came across a cart loaded with wheat, with its wheels sunk deep in the muddy road. With his powerful arms, he helped the driver move the cart out of the rut, to the amazement of all standers-by. Since then he had been known far and near as "iron-armed hero."

In 1913, at a marketplace in a neighboring

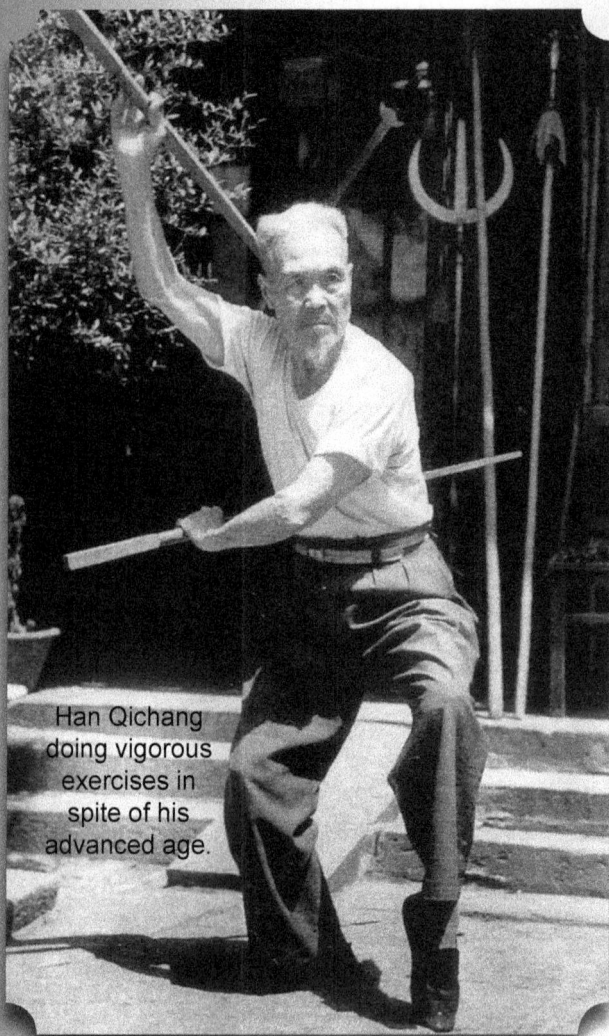

Han Qichang doing vigorous exercises in spite of his advanced age.

village, Han happened to see a wushu routine with a variety of movements and postures, some as quiet as those of a gentle maid and some as swift as those of a running rabbit. After many inquiries, he got the performer's address and came to his home. It was none other than Yun Meichi, a grand master of the ancient wushu school called "Plum-Flower Pegs" done while walking on pegs in the form of a plum flower petal.

Dropping on his knees, Han kowtowed to Yun again and again, requesting to be accepted as a disciple. To test the applicant's

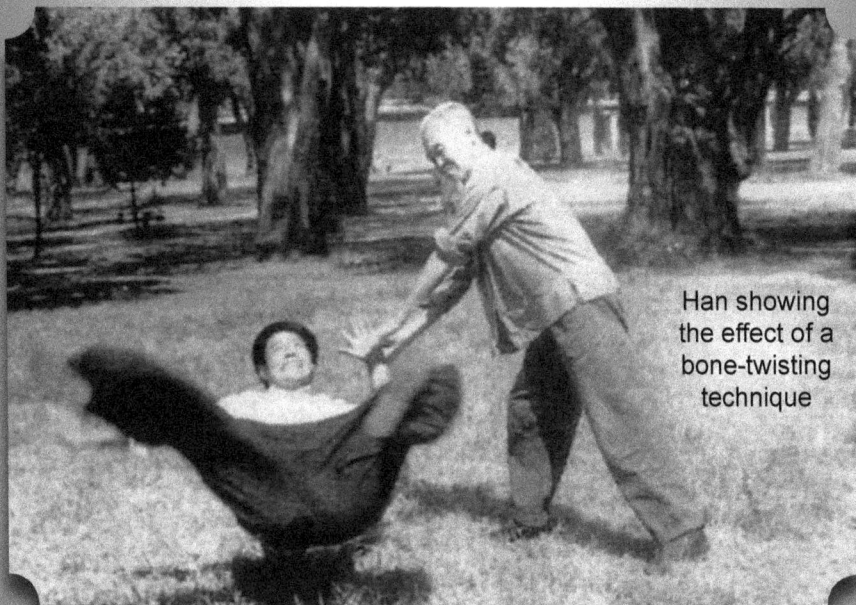

Han showing
the effect of a
bone-twisting
technique

strength, the master told his youngest son to try a bout with Han.
At the sight of a small boy much shorter than himself, Han thought
gleefully that he was sure to win. But he was knocked down before
he knew it. After losing several bouts, Han had to admit defeat,
thinking that the "plum-flower-pegs" could really work miracles.

It was four miles to the Yun's. For three long years Han would go
there every day, until he had acquired the basic skills, which he later
improved under the tutelage of another famous master named Zhao
Yinglian. It was not long before Han established himself as a wushu
master.

In 1917, there was a big flood on the Xutuo River, causing a famine
to Shenxian and other counties. Han was obliged to go to Tianjin
and then to Baoding where, on his former master Broadsword
Li's recommendation, he earned a living as a wushu instructor at
military barracks. At the same time, he made a name for himself
by winning many challenge contests as a representative of Hebei
Province.

In 1933, he went to Beijing, where he taught wushu for some years
at middle schools and founded the Jianzhu Martial Art Society as
training center of the Plum-Flower Pegs exercises.

49

Han never showed off his skills and was highly respected by his colleagues and followers for his modesty and kind-heartedness. When he was engaged at Zicheng Middle School, some trouble makers challenged him. To avoid hurting them and save their face, he just leaned quietly against a tree, holding a thick branch in his hands. When the first challenger came up to him, a cracking sound was heard from where Han stood. The branch was seen in two pieces. All the adversaries sneaked away in fear and shame, knowing better than to take him on.

Han was best known for his single-minded devotion to wushu. He has spent his whole life practicing and teaching it, without stopping for a single day until he drew his last breath at the age of 94.

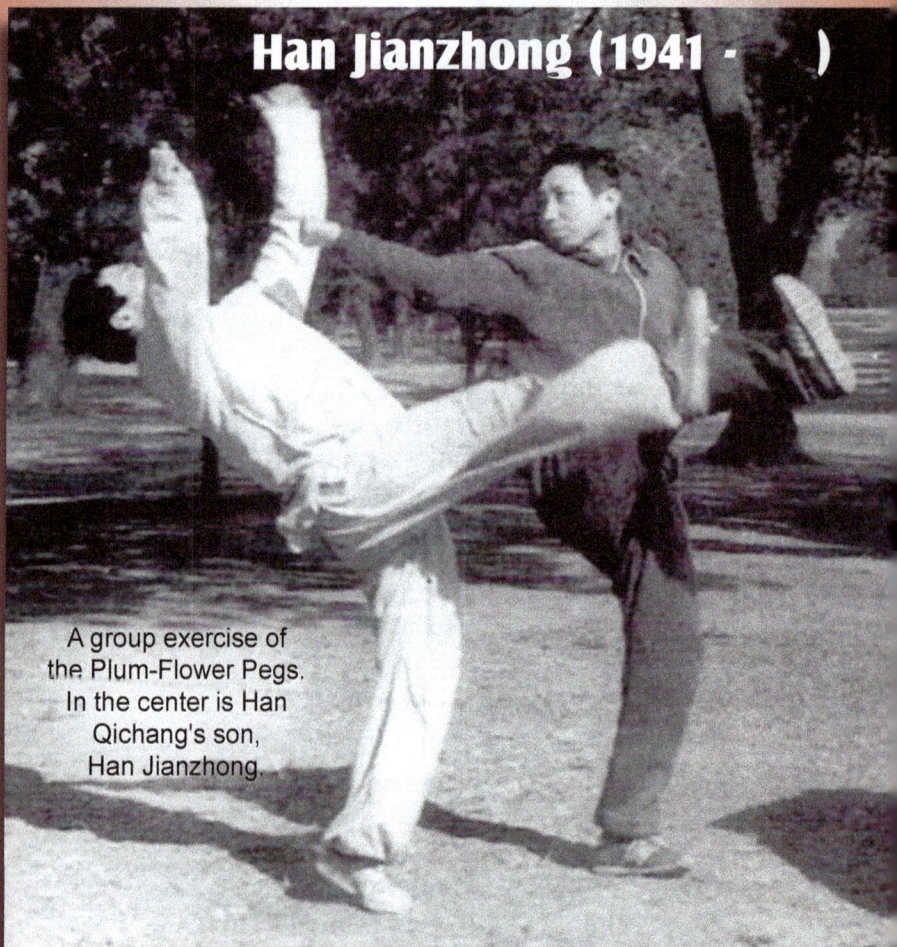

Han Jianzhong (1941 -)

A group exercise of the Plum-Flower Pegs. In the center is Han Qichang's son, Han Jianzhong.

Master Han Jianzhong

Han Jianzhong, head of the wushu teaching group at the China People's Police University, has inherited everything about the "Plum-Flower Pegs" from his father Han Qichang, founder of this particular school - including routines combined with qigong and forms practiced with long spear and "spring and autumn" broadsword. Besides, he is a master of the cheng, gong, and ying schools and the author of several books about "Plum-Flower Pegs" exercises and more than 60 theses on traditional Chinese martial arts.

Han is as faithful to his friends and all honest people as he is intolerant with wrong-doers. Using his excellent kungfu, he has vanquished armed thugs with his bare hands. Owing to his fruitful work in education and research, he is highly respected by his colleagues and followers at home and abroad and has won a series of honours and positions: National Outstanding Wushu Instructor in 1983, Secretary-General of Beijing Plum-Flower Pegs Society and member of the Beijing Wushu Association in 1984, and in 1985, consultant of a society setup by Shaolin Temple in Henan Province. In recognition of his outstanding achievements, this society has conferred on him a flag inscribed with the words: "Cream of Martial Arts" - praise he adequately deserves.

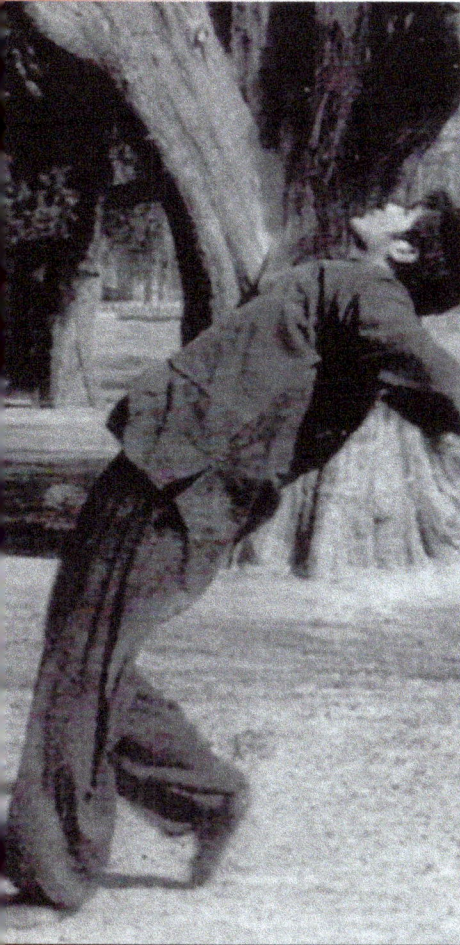

Forms of Plum Flower Pegs

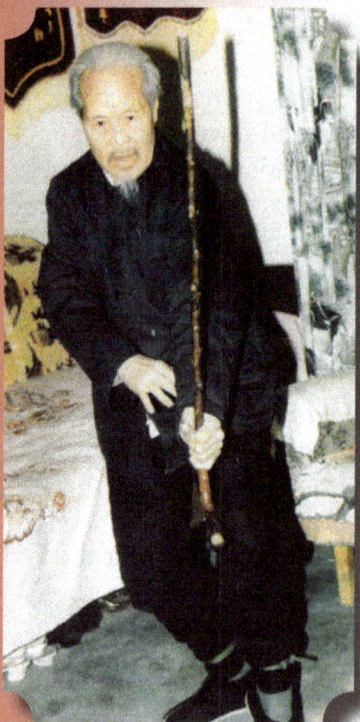

Han Qichang

The "Plum-Flower Peg" exercises, also known as "plum-flower" boxing, are done on wooden pegs. Now they are sometimes practiced on flat ground. Hence another name of "fallen plum-flower" exercises.

This school of wushu may be traced back to the 17th century, when it was rooted among the common folk in Henan, Hebei and Shandong Provinces in the lower reaches of the Yellow River. It has been handed down from generation to generation first as an heirloom and then, from the 1740s onward, also outside family clans. In the comtemporary period, the best-known master of this school was Han Qichang (1894 - 1988).

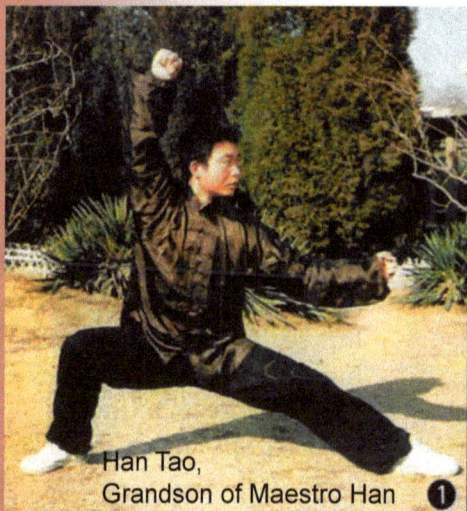

Han Tao,
Grandson of Maestro Han ❶

The school is divided into big frame and small frame styles with five different forms, namely, 1) the big form, or "the red phoenix facing the sun"; 2) the follow through form, or "the big roc spreading its wings"; 3) the twisted form, or "the peddler carrying two hills on his shoulder pole"; 4) the small form, or "the monkey climbing tree branches"; 5) the beaten form, or "King

Xiangyu dismantling his armour". These forms may be alternated in exercises.

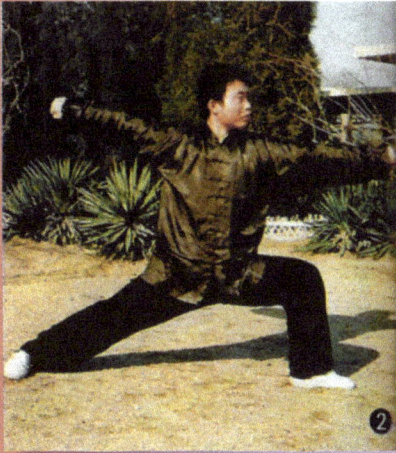

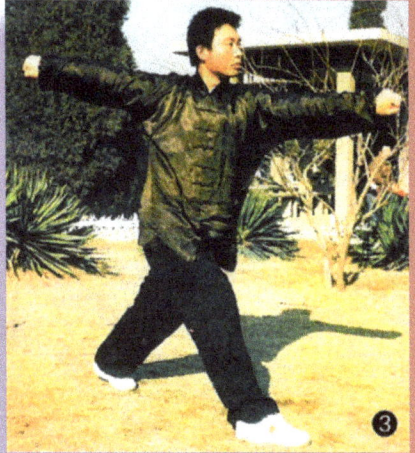

The footwork consists of the "eight-direction" steps and walking steps. The former is also called "chun bu" or "varying steps", which are subdivided into the fundamental "small steps" used in dodging, turning and attacking, and the middle and big steps, both used

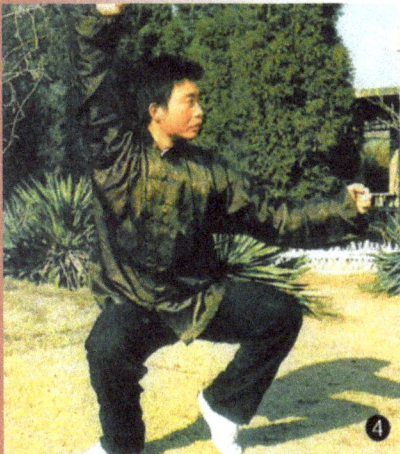

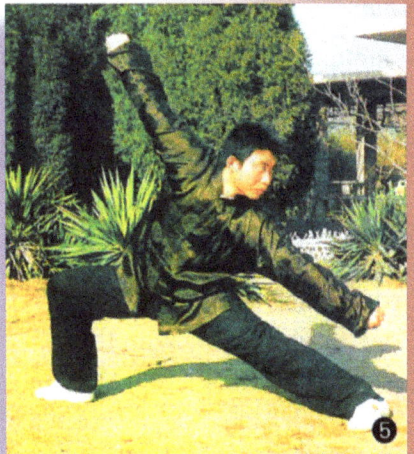

against more than one adversary from an advantageous position requiring fast yet well-controlled speed, agility in charges and retreats, changes in different situations, coordination with rises and falls of the body, and harmony between motion and stillness. The walking steps are subdivided into the swaying step, the thrusting step and the retreating step.

The most popular routines with weapons are the Play with broadsword, exercises with long spear in 12 forms and hitting methods with long cudgel. Other long weapons used include the halbert, shuo (a long handled spear), dang (a kind of fork), rake-shaped ba, hooked spear and long pole. Among the short weapons mention may be made of sword, broadsword with rings, tiger-headed hook and crescent dagger, and meteor hammer.

The pegs are usually of wood, projecting about 1.1 meter above the ground, 1 meter apart from another lengthwise and 0.5 meter breadthwise. Their height is increased with technical proficiency. Sometimes bricks are used, first lying flat, then on the side and finally on the end to raise the degree of difficulty.

The exercises are done in different patterns such as the Big Dipper, Three Stars, Eight-Diagrams, the Five Elements (metal, wood, water, fire and earth), and Nine Squares - all based on the principle of harmonization with the celestial phenomena above, with the 24 divisions of the solar year in the middle and, down below, with the 12 Earthly Branches used in combination with the Heavenly Stems to designate years, months, days and hours. Movements high above the ground require an upright body posture and make the exercises all the more difficult. The practice suits group exercises in

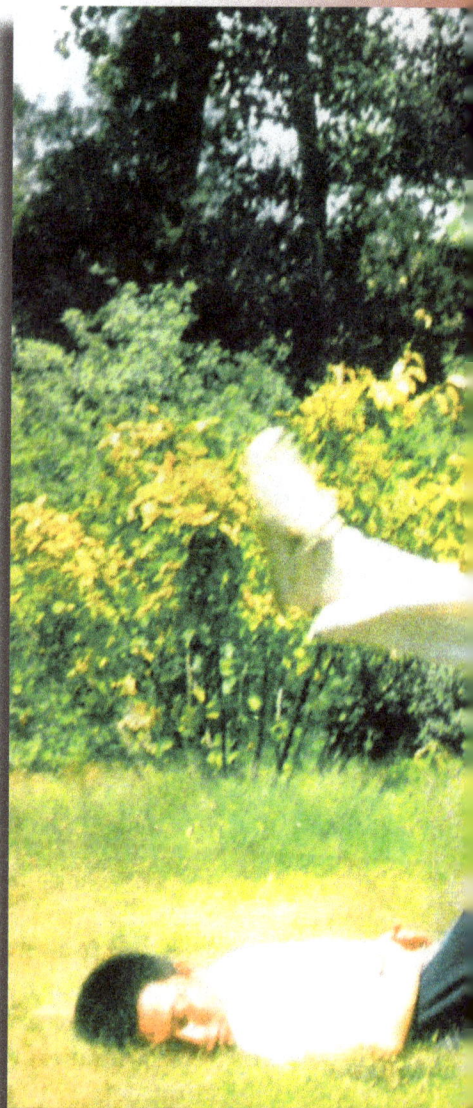

which the individuals are formed into the shape of a plum flower now opening and now closing its petals. Patterns may change and vary at the group's fancy, so long as the movements are fluent, orderly and free from monotony.

The training starts with the five basic forms aimed to acquire fighting skills and coordinated abdominal breathing. Constant practice helps to improve reflexes and senses of stability and precision, increase muscular strength and elasticity, promote cardio-pulmonary function and raise one's fitness level as a whole.

Han Jianzhong

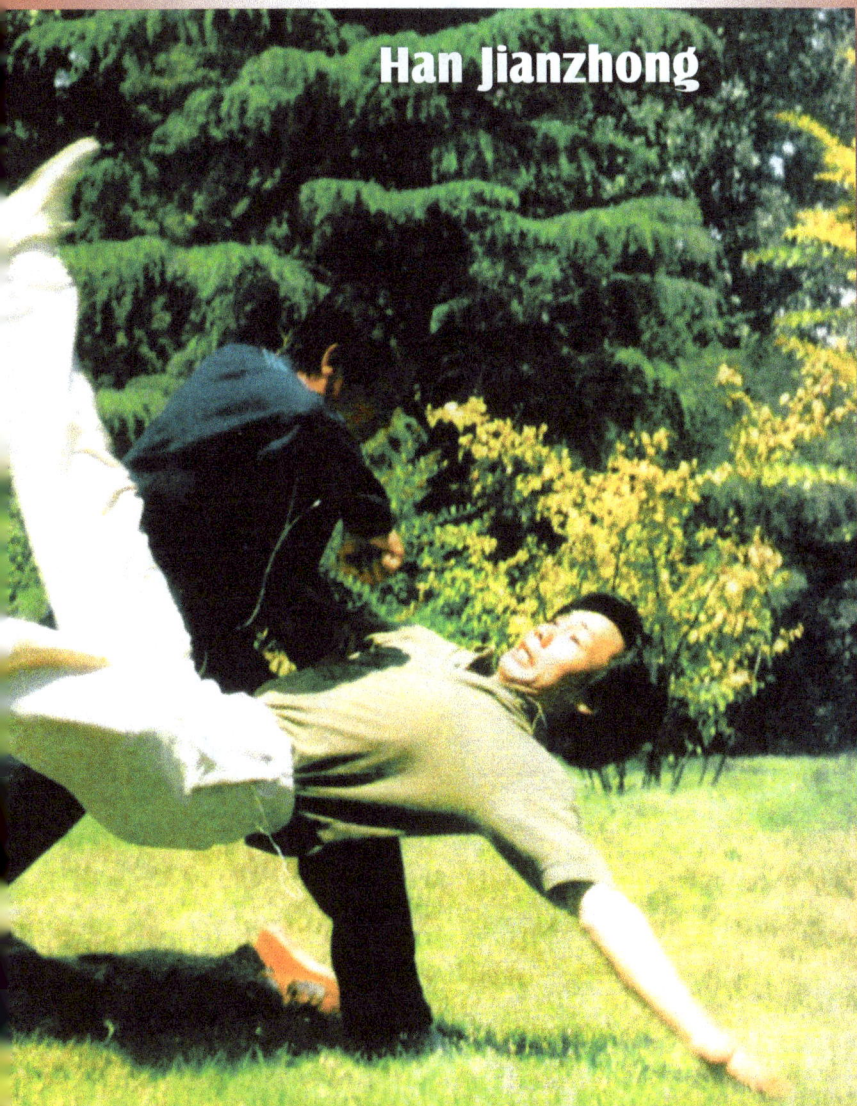

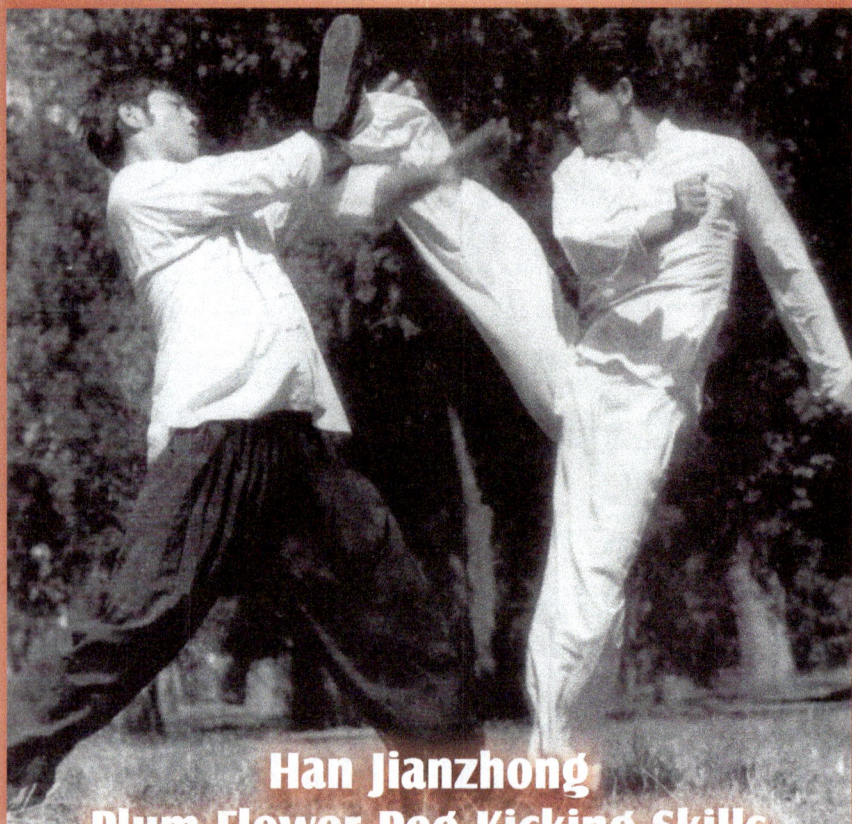

Han Jianzhong
Plum Flower Peg Kicking Skills

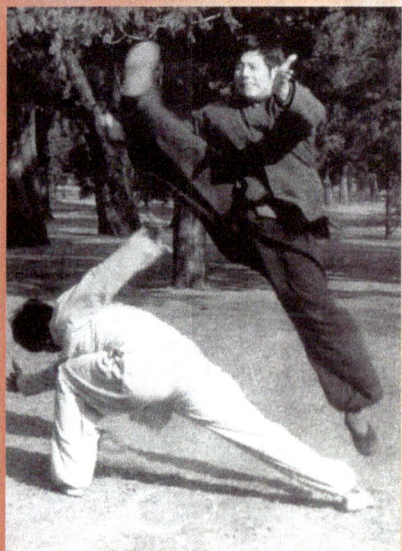

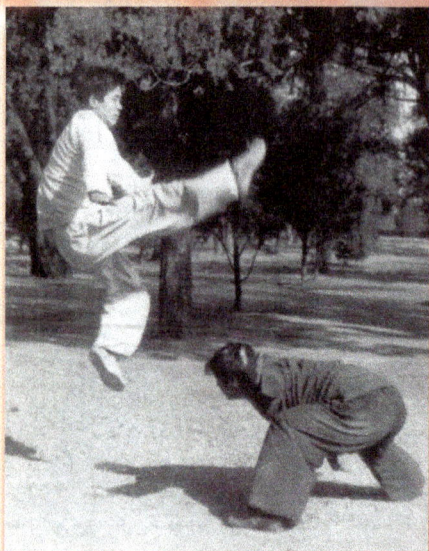

NATURAL BOXING

Zi Ran Men: The Natural School

The Natural School is based on an abstruse philosophy as can be seen from its guiding principles: "There is neither beginning for mobility and immobility nor end to changes. The movements, whether solid or void, are done naturally."

As pointed out by Wan Laisheng, a wushu master who inherited the Natural School from his grandfather, everything will come to you naturally, through a training that "makes your hands as soft as cotton and your trunk as hard as iron," that "enables you to fight without being seen by your opponent" and "makes you look like a baby, from whose blows no one can escape unscathed." There are more than 30 kinds of weapons used in the training, including yuanyang huan (mandarin duck rings), zimuqiu (son-and-mother balls), tiesha bao (iron sand bag) and hukou bang (tiger-mouth cudgel).

The Natural School is said to have been created by an eccentric wushu master nicknamed Dwarf Xu who lived towards the end of

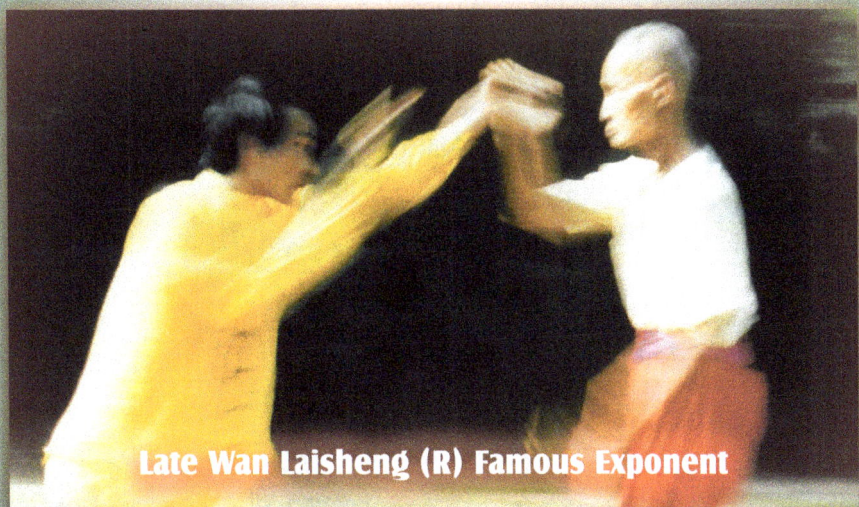

Late Wan Laisheng (R) Famous Exponent

the Qing Dynasty (1644-1911), by absorbing the essence of many schools on the basis of Taoist theories. During the past century or so, it has been handed down exclusively through three generations of three families, namely, Dwarf Xu, Du Xinwu and Wan Laisheng.

While emphasizing on internal work, the Natural School is also aimed at fighting skills and characterized by simple yet hard training. The routine is free from all superfluous movements as contained in many other schools for the mere purpose of performance and demonstration. Instead of relying on a few fortes, it attaches great importance to the substantial training of jing, qi and shen (essence, energy, and vitality) and a full mobilization of the whole body, including the limbs, the trunk, the head and neck and the joints.

The routine includes both defensive and offensive movements, long-range kicks in attack as well short parries in defence. As a motto goes, you must know how to shrink like a crane, strike like a thunderbolt, move about like an ape and turn round like a millstone. Another watchword: Create something out of nothing and do everything at your free will.

A practitioner of the Natural School must always be on the alert and keep doing sparring exercises with his master to get the hang of the basics. As a result of the combination of internal and external work and of mobility and immobility, and with all actions following a natural course, he will become stronger and stronger both physically and mentally until the attainment of perfection in body and mind.

Below: A chief exponent of the Natural School was 87-year-old Wan Laisheng who lived in the coastal city of Fuzhou.

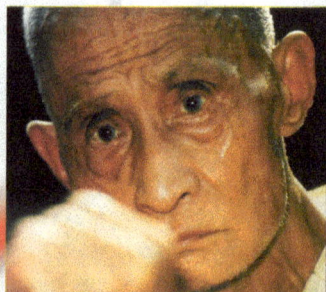

Du Xin Wu
Standard for the Natural School
(1869 - 1953)

Du Xinwu, a well known master of
the Natural School, was born in Zili
County, Hunan Province. He began to
learn wushu at the age of six when he
was studying at a private school. Three
years later, he was fortunate enough to
be apprenticed to Yan Ke, a scholar of
literature and martial arts. The clever
boy made rapid progress and found no
peer in his native town at the age of 10.

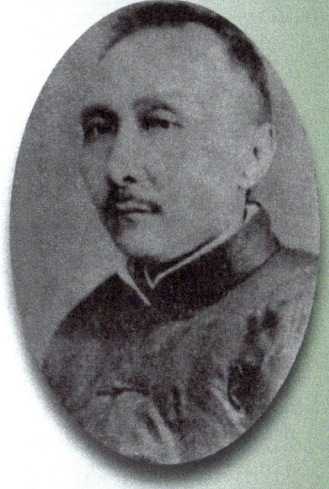

Then his master was confined to bed and
Du Xinwu went into the hills of Gazi
Mountain, where he met an old Taoist,
one of Yan Ke's friends. The Taoist was
said to have the habit of jumping over a gateless high fence when he
went into and came out of his homestead. He passed on his wushu
skills to Du.

At the age of 13, Du was introduced to an eccentric person named
Dwarf Xu, also known as "Strange Hero South of the Yangtze," who
hailed from Guizhou Province and was wandering from one place
to another.

Thinking Du to be a prodigy, Dwarf Xu taught him everything
about the Natural School he had founded, including the feat of
"light footwork," which enabled him to jump over three tables
placed atop of each other.

In 1885, when he was 16 years of age, Du Xinwu accompanied
his master to Guizhou and Sichuan and broadened his vision
through contacts with famous wushu maestros of different schools.
Seeing that he had reached maturity, Dwarf Xu left him all on his
own. Two years later, Du tried to find a job in an escort bureau

in Sichuan. At the sight of his small size, the hefty director made little of him and challenged him to a bout. Du gave him three "sweeping kicks" and threw him to the ground, unable to get up for a counterattack. Du was accepted as an escort. He carried out all his missions successfully and struck terror into the highwaymen's hearts. But he grew tired of the job and returned to his home town two years later.

In 1900, Du Xinwu went to study in Japan. While aboard a ship just leaving the dock in Shanghai, he saw a boat catching up in the wake, calling the ship to stop to pick up a Chinese merchant's trunk which had been left behind. But the haughty captain paid no heed to it. In great indignation, Du jumped into the boat and back on board ship with the trunk, which he handed to its owner as many passengers looked at him in no small wonder.

Du Xinwu entered the Imperial University, majoring in agriculture. Relying on his unusual fighting skills, he revenged some insults done to his fellow countrymen and no one dared to ride roughshod over them again when he was nearby.

In 1905, when the China Revolutionary League was founded under the leadership of Sun Yat-sen, Du Xinwu joined it at the recommendation of his classmate Song Jiaoren and took charge of the founder's safety. After the Revolution of 1911 put an end to the Qing Dynasty, Du was appointed councillor of the Ministry of Agriculture and Forestry headed by Song Jiaoren and engaged as a professor of an agricultural institute.

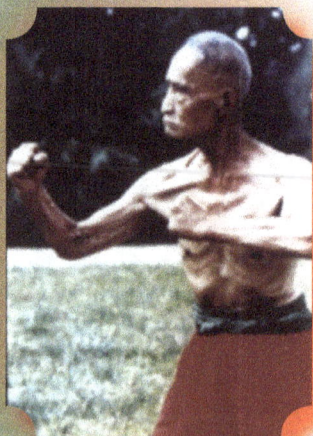

During Du's stay in Beijing, he accepted Wan Laisheng (left) and Guo Qifeng as his disciples of wushu. When receiving his second disciple, he gave a demonstration of his "light footwork" by performing a dazzling Natural School routine as he walked a dozen rounds or so on the edge of a big round cauldron. His pupil kowtowed to him again and again after he landed gently on the ground without panting or showing the slightest sign of fatigue.

After the central government moved to Nanjing in 1927, Du Xinwu worked in the Ministry of Agriculture and Mining and then as Deputy Director of an experimental farm in Henan Province. In 1932, he was invited to sit on a panel of jury for the Second National Wushu Contest held in Changsha, capital of Hunan Province.

He retired in 1949 to a peaceful life in his birthplace, living together with his daughter's family. Still he kept the honorable post of advisor to the provincial people's government until his death at 84. Watch for stories of Du's heroic martial arts exploits in a separate volume of *Grandmaster's of China* book.

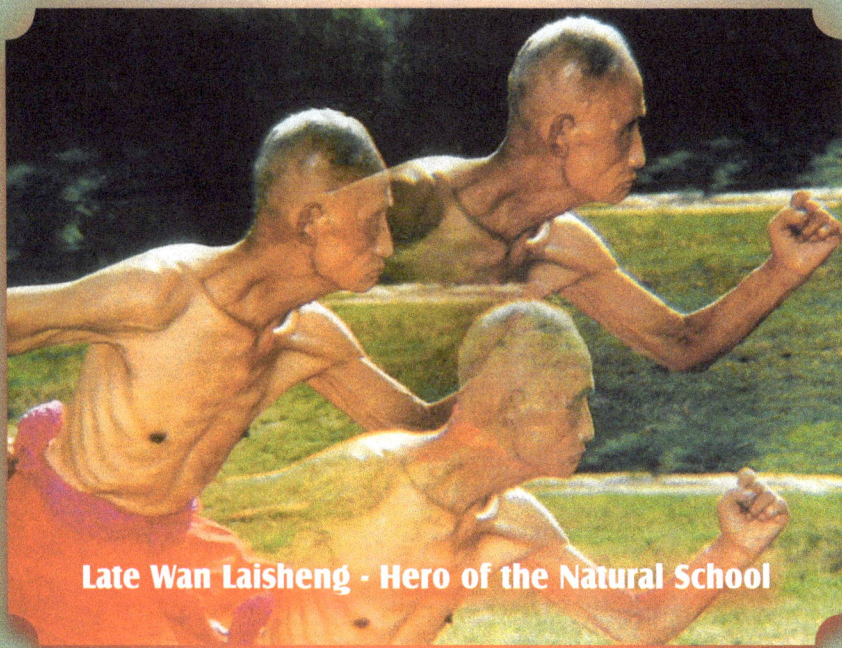

Late Wan Laisheng - Hero of the Natural School

Sidelight

Late in 1929, Du Xinwu was invited to officiate a national wushu contest which was held in Hangzhou, capital of Zhejiang Province, and lasted for a whole month. At the closing ceremony, the audience asked him to demonstrate his Natural Gate school skills in fleet-footed circular walk, for which he had been known as "Quick Fairy." Finding it hard to turn down the insistent request, he stepped on the stage. To warm himself up, he walked round and round like an ordinary man. The spectators were disappointed and started booing when he quickened his steps until he looked like a whirlwind - eerie, shapeless and roaring as if it were going to tear down the roof. Then he came to a sudden stop, a calm smile on his face and without panting or showing the least sign of fatigue. In answer to the audience's encores, he repeated his performance - this time on his tiptoes!

61

Wan Laisheng

(1903 - 1992)

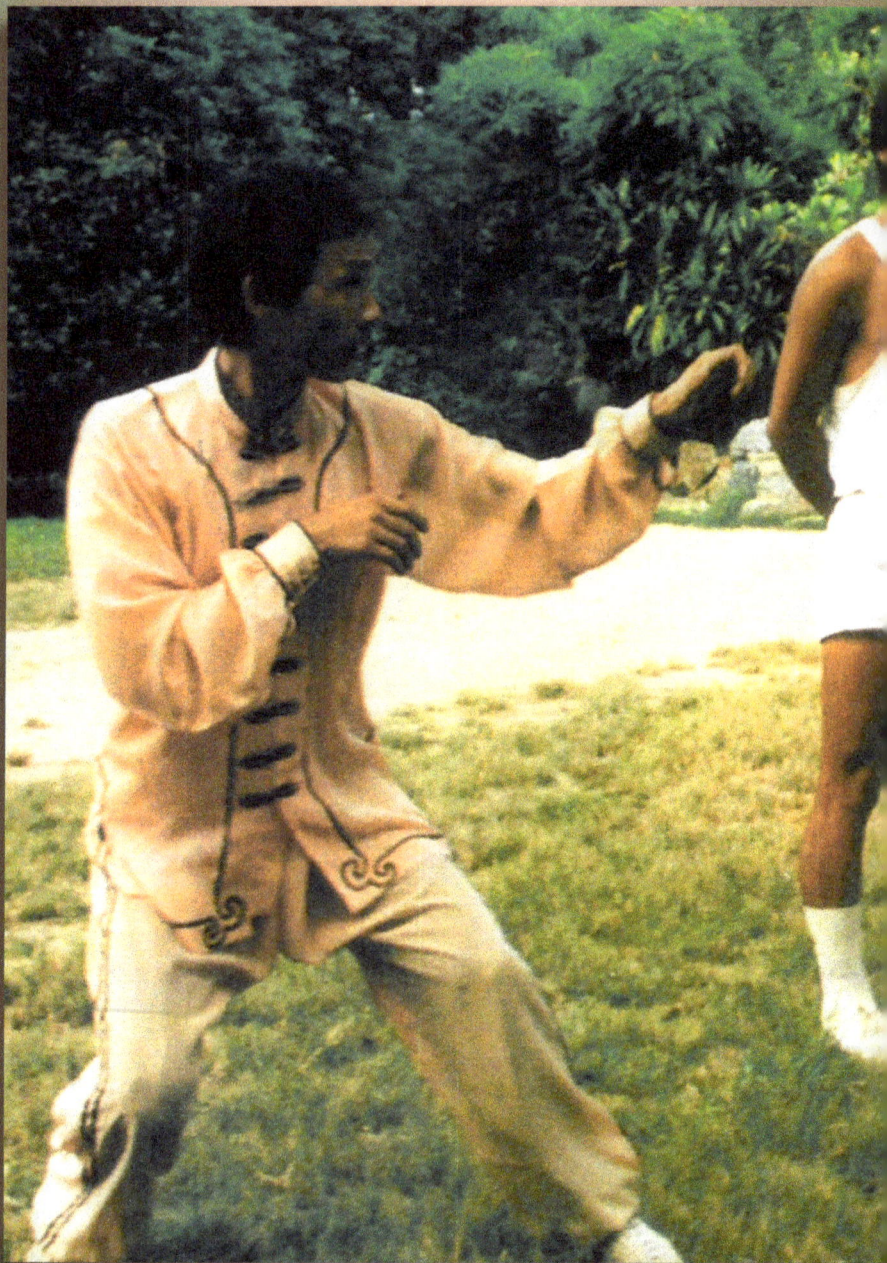

Wan Laisheng, alias Wan Changqing, was born into a scholar's family in Wuchang. At the age of 17, he went to Beijing to study at the Forestry Department of the National Agricultural University. There he made the

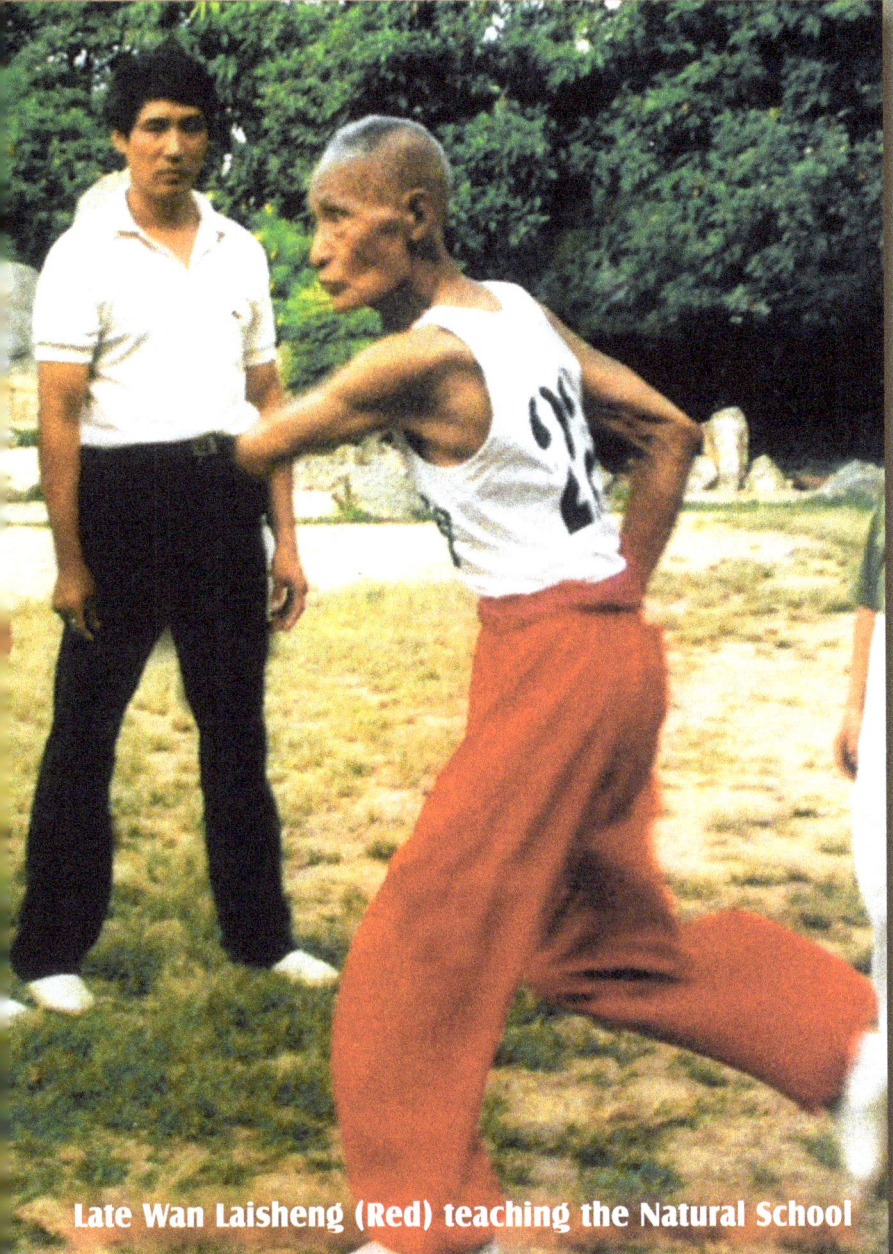

Late Wan Laisheng (Red) teaching the Natural School

63

acquaintance of Zhao Xinzhou, head of the Ever-Victorious Escort Bureau, who undertook to teach him the Liuhe (six-in-one) exercises of the Shaolin School.

After graduating with distinction, he stayed at the Agricultural University as a faculty member and continued his studies of wushu under as many masters as he could get access to in the city.

Hearing that Du Xinwu, an expert of the Natural School, was working with the Ministry of Agriculture and Mining in Beijing, Wan implored him time and again to teach him the art. Moved by his sincerity and seeing that he had a good command of the basic skills of wushu, Du accepted him as his first disciple. It was after seven years of hard work that Wan finally mastered the theories and practice of the Natural School.

Afterwards, he broadened his store of knowledge with other schools like form-and-will, eight-diagram, taiji, monkey, pigua, arhat and southern exercises he picked up from well known masters like Liu Baichuan, Wang Xiangzhai and Wang Rongbiao. At the same time, at the request of the editor-in-chief of *Chen Bao (Morning News)*, he contributed a series of articles on his views of the different wushu schools, which were published in 1928 in a 200,000-worded book under the title of *A Collection of Reviews on Wushu*, the first treatise in modern times. It was the first time he used the pen name of Wan Laisheng, by which he was known until now.

In the same year, Wan participated in the First National Wushu Contest with credits, thus earning a nationwide reputation that brought in a flood of letters asking him to teach wushu. Together with his cousin Wan Laiping and three of his colleagues Gu Ruzhang, Li Xianwu and Fu Zhensong, he went to Guangzhou where he accepted the post of director of the Guangdong-Guangxi Wushu Academy - an event that has gone down in China's history of wushu as "five tigers going south."

In the 1930s, Wan Laisheng travelled to many other places - to Changsha where he acted as director of the Hunan Wushu Institute in 1931, to Hong Kong where he supervised a wushu tournament in 1933, and to Guilin where he was put in charge of the Physical Education Department of Guangxi University in 1934, and to

Fujian where he founded the Yong'an Teachers School for Physical Education in 1939. From 1944 onward he taught at the Fujian Agricultural College as a professor of sports until his retirement in 1951. Even afterwards he devoted much of his time to orthopaedics.

Wan Laisheng has brought up a few generations of wushu masters and written 16 books, including *Illustrated Arhat Exercises of the Shaolin School*, *The Cream of Wushu*, *Traditional Chinese Orthopaedics*, *The Natural School of Wushu*, *Talks on Wushu* and *Spearplay in 24 Forms*.

Up until his passing in 1992, he worked in a number of posts: Member of the Fujian Chinese People's Political Consultative Conference, Honorary President of the Fujian Wushu Association, Honorary Director of Wanlu Wushu Academy in Xiamen and Fuzhou Wushu Academy, advisor of Wudang Boxing Society in Hubei Province, general advisor of Taiyuan Natural School Society in Shanxi Province and professor emeritus of the Lanting Institute.

In his own words, he has devoted his whole life to four things, that is, traditional Chinese medicine, practice and teaching of traditional Chinese martial arts, and writing books on these subjects. And he was particularly happy that the Natural School of wushu had been carried on at home and abroad by scores of his disciples.

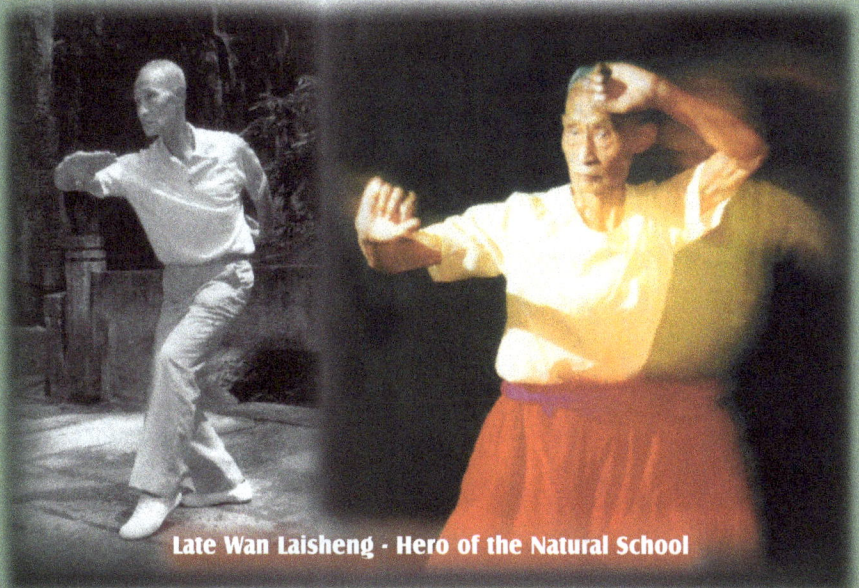

Late Wan Laisheng · Hero of the Natural School

DACHENG BOXING

Creating New from the Old

The name of this kind of exercise implies a combination of some major wushu schools. It has but a history of little more than half a century, dating back to the 1940s when it was initiated by Wang Xiangzhai, a famous master in Beijing, who had learned form-and-will exercises from Guo Yunshen and travelled widely along the Yangtze River to study other schools.

In the early '20s, when Wang was teaching in Shanghai, he found out

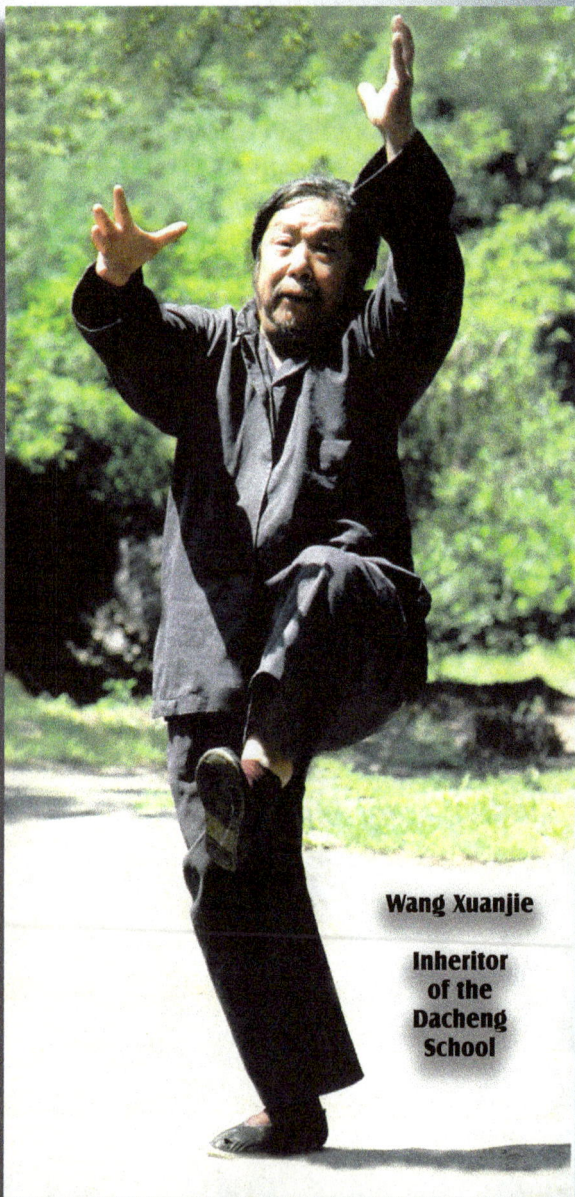

Wang Xuanjie

Inheritor of the Dacheng School

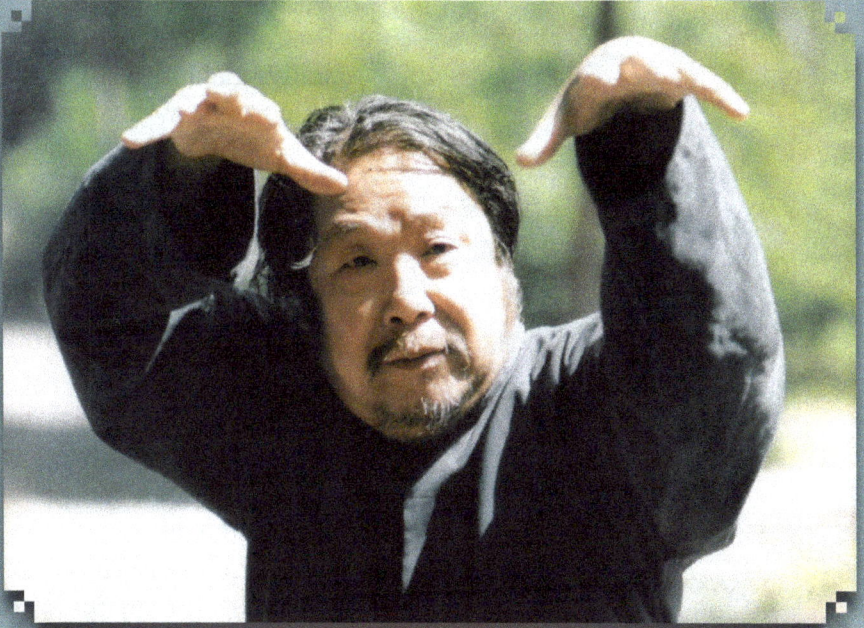

that many of his disciples were mainly concerned with the form of exercises to the neglect of "will". That's putting the cart before the horse, he thought to himself. So he changed the name of "form-and-will" into "will", emphasizing that one should pay more attention to the mental aspect instead of limiting oneself to the physical aspect. "Put more spirit into your movements," he told his pupils. "Don't seek after the superficial."

After some time, the master found some pupils going to the other extremity - an over emphasis on the mental aspect to the neglect of physical training. It dawned upon him that he must have over stretched his point in changing the name. He made another extensive journey in the country and came into contact with many wushu masters, resulting in a considerable improvement in his own theoretical understanding and training methods. Casting away the usual bias towards other schools and absorbing their best elements, he worked out a new routine based mainly on standing exercises and without a set pattern for movements - a routine he called "dacheng".

Dacheng is quite different from the "will" boxing he had been

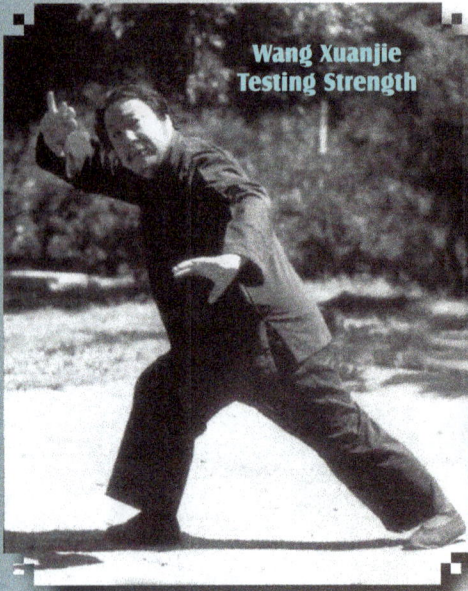

Wang Xuanjie
Testing Strength

teaching, which was basically a variety of the traditional form-and-will school, only with a stress, or too much stress, on the mental activity in the exercises. Dacheng, on the other hand, pays equal attention to six things, namely; the spirit, form, consciousness, strength, vital energy and skills.

While adopting the basic training methods used in the form-and-will exercises, the new "Dacheng" also assimilated some from the Shaolin School in transcendental meditation, from the Taiji School in the cultivation of vital energy and from the "Eight-Diagram Palm" School in body position and footwork. Thus it has developed into a unique style and marked a great improvement in the theory and practice of traditional martial arts.

In doing the Dacheng exercises, one should "prevent the spirit from overflowing, the will from showing outside, the form from hurting the body and the strength from going beyond the extremities, while keeping energy flowing through the whole body and the methods in harmony with nature." Based on standing exercises, the movements should be performed with increased tempo and amount

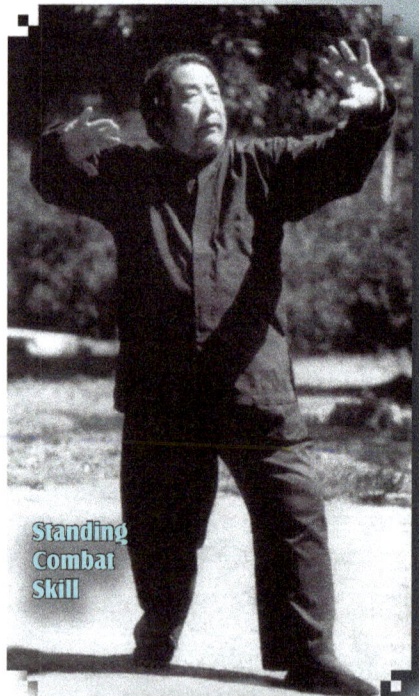

Standing
Combat
Skill

of physical exertion in the whole training period, always maintaining unity among the above-mentioned six respects.

There are seven skills in the exercises:

1) Standing skill: This is subdivided into skill for the purpose of raising fitness level through relaxation and tranquillity, and the skill for the purpose of combat.

2) Testing strength: All the standing exercises are coordinated with auxiliary skills to mobilize internal strength for outward movements.

A Form of Footwork

3) Footwork: This is an application of internal strength to the movements of lower limbs, such as shuffling steps.

4) Explosive force: Movements are brought to a sudden stop.

5) Utterance of sounds: This is used together with explosive force to accentuate power and momentum.

6) Pushing hands: An exercise between two partners.

7) Practical combat: This is sometimes called "duanshou," meaning "breaking hands".

The seven skills form an organic whole and are indispensable in both training and actual fighting.

Dacheng School is an important development of wushu theories and training methods, combining health-building and martial art in a set of simple and highly efficient exercises, as is clearly distinguished from routines of other schools.

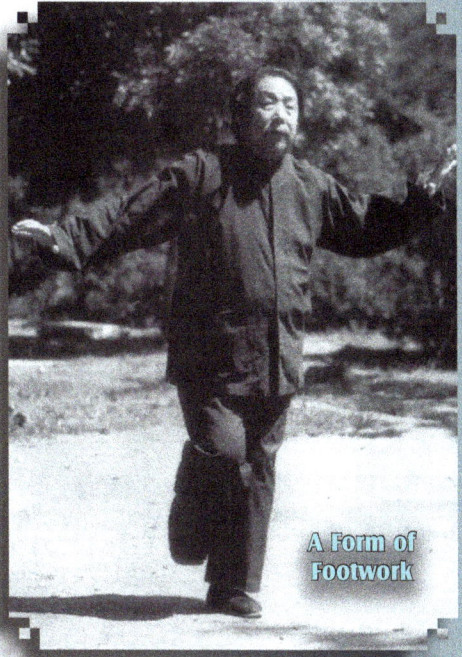

Wang Xiangzhai

Blending Many Schools

(1885 - 1963)

Wang Xiangzhai, alias Wang Yuzeng, was born in Weilin Village, Shenxian County, Hebei Province. He began learning wushu at the age of 14, which improved his poor health and enabled him to live to an age of 78.

He was first apprenticed to Guo Yunshen, a wushu master versed in the form-and-will school, who loved the bright boy so much that he passed on all his skills to him, thus laying a groundwork for his future career.

Wang Xiangzhai

In 1907, Wang set out on an extensive travel until he settled down in Beijing six years later. While serving as a wushu instructor in one of Yuan Shikai's army units, he had the opportunity of learning a lot from his colleagues Shang Yunxiang, Sun Lutang and Liu Wenhua, all masters of nation-wide renown. From 1918, he travelled to Hunan, Hubei, Shaanxi, Anhui, Zhejiang and Fujian Provinces where he called on many big shots in the wushu community, including some monks and abbots of Shaolin Monastery in the Songshan Mountains and Xie Tiefu, known as Boxer No. 1 south of the Yangtze River, with whom he built lasting friendships.

Thus Wang acquired a wide store of knowledge of the different schools of wushu, which he made full use of and created the "will" boxing characterized by concentration and naturalness instead of

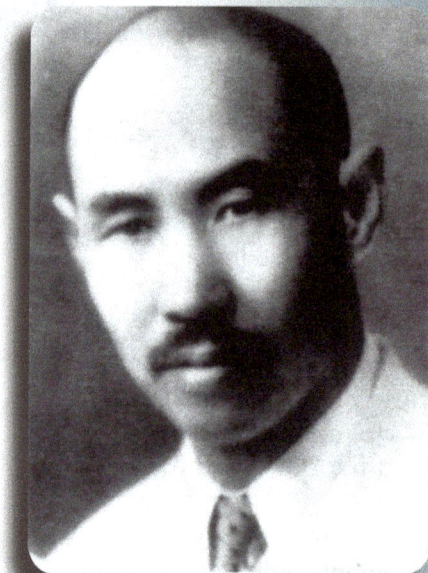

one-sided emphasis on physical exercises. In 1940, some of Wang's friends suggested that he change the name into "Dacheng", meaning "a combination of many schools". The new name was accepted and spread far and wide, especially after some articles were published in the newspapers *Truth* and *New People*.

Wang had to receive an endless stream of visitors coming from various parts of the country and abroad. A world boxing champion in lightweight class from Hungary made a challenge to Wang and was defeated. He wrote an article entitled "*Chinese Martial Art as I See It*", in which he spoke highly of Wang. Among Wang's guests were also top notch Japanese judoists and swordsmen who praised his unusual combat skills after measuring strength with him. Hong Xuru, a well-known master in Beijing, lost all his three bouts with Wang and brought his disciples to him to learn the Dacheng boxing skills.

In 1947, Wang set up an academy at the Imperial Ancestral Temple in Beijing as a training centre of standing exercises. In 1950, he was put in charge of the wushu section of the All-China Sports Federation then in the preparatory phase. In the next year, he was invited to teach standing exercises at the Hebei Traditional Chinese Medicine Research Institute in Baoding, where he made an extensive study of the therapeutical value of wushu. His research exerted a deep influence on health work.

Wang wrote two books, *The Essentials of Will Boxing* and *On Dacheng Boxing*, and a number of theses in which he put forth the theories of his school with great depth of thought. One authoritative exponent of this school was Wang Xuanjie, the last and perhaps best disciple of founder, Wang Xiangzhai.

Wang Xuanjie

Weakling to Dacheng Grandmaster

(1932 - 2000)

Born into a scholarly family in Beijing, Wang Xuanjie was a weakling in childhood. He took up wushu in order to improve his health, without knowing that he would become a famous master in the future. Fortunately, he had the opportunity of learning from a few good masters - Abbot Yue Lang of Hua Yan Temple who taught him the art of transcendental meditation, qigong and acupuncture; He Dequan distinguished for his kicking skills; and Xiong Deshan, a national wrestling champion in the '30s.

Then he spent three years learning the Dacheng School from Li Yunzeng and Yang Demao, both disciples of its founder Wang Xiangzhai. He became physically strong and technically proficient.

In the late '50s, Wang Xuanjie often went to Zhongshan park to practice wushu together with other enthusiasts. His talent came to the notice of Wang Xiangzhai, who was pushing 70 and wanted to choose someone as the genuine inheritor of his Dacheng School of martial arts. Wang Xuanjie proved to be the best choice.

Under the old master's tutelage, Wang Xuanjie made such rapid progress that he defeated a number of well-known martial artists - taiji boxers Li Fushou and Gao Yuqing, kicking expert Wu Changyin, national wrestling champion Li Liugeng in middleweight class, and Thai-style boxer Liu Sheng from Hong Kong. What's more important, he has brought up a host of masters who, like himself, used to be of feeble constitution and have borne out the undisputed value of Dacheng exercises not only as a unique form of wushu, but also as a means to raise one's fitness level.

Wang wholeheartedly dedicated himself to the cause of wushu until he passed in March of 2000, from a heart attack.

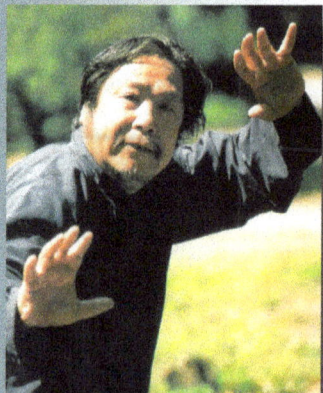

Wang
Xuanjie

Second
Generation
Dacheng
Boxing

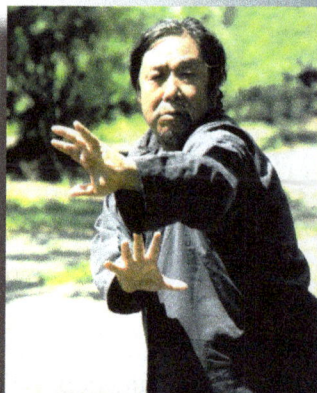

EIGHT-DIAGRAM PALM BOXING

From Taoist Enlightenment

The "Eight Diagrams," which first appeared in the Chinese classic *Book of Changes*, are each composed of three horizontal lines - either whole or broken in the middle - imposed one upon another, as symbols of the eight natural phenomena, namely, the heaven, earth, thunder, wind, rivers, fire, mountains and lakes. They are often placed around a yin-yang circle halved by a line of "s" with a dot inside the two curves - as a symbol of "taiji" or the universe. The whole picture embodies the main ideas of Taoist philosophy, which regards the heaven and earth as the chief sources of all natural and social phenomena.

The Eight-Diagram palm is a kind of wushu exercise with the palms changing in

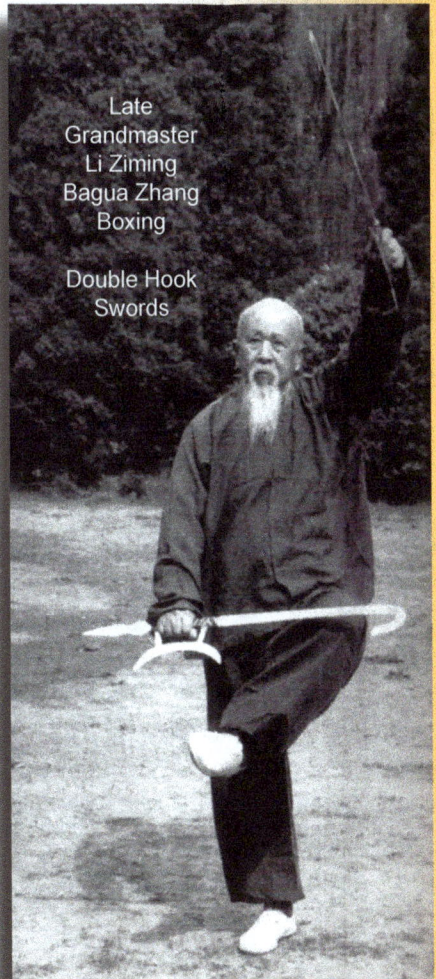

Late Grandmaster Li Ziming Bagua Zhang Boxing

Double Hook Swords

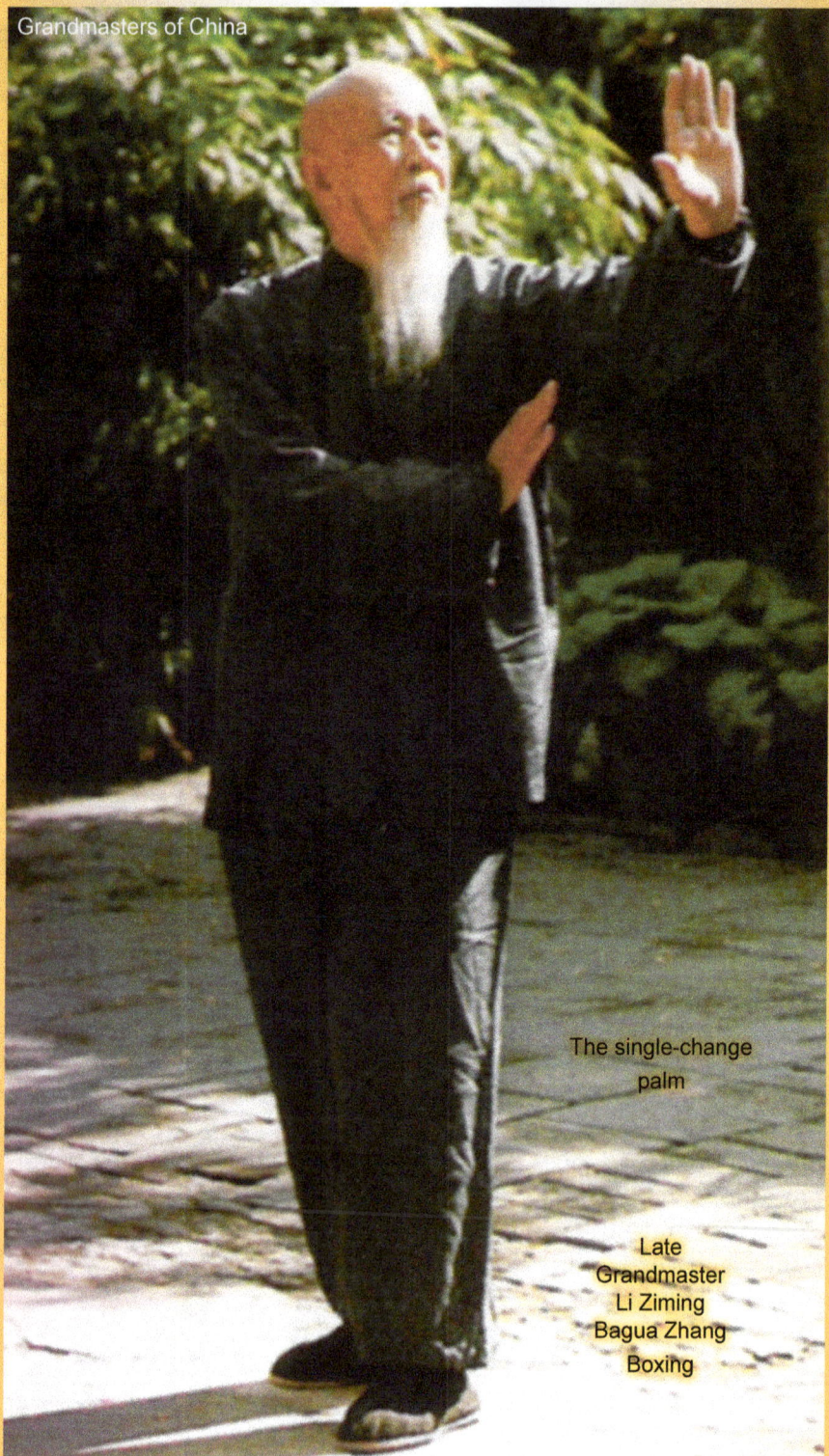

The single-change palm

Late Grandmaster Li Ziming Bagua Zhang Boxing

form and position and the feet moving in a circular path, as though around the circle of taiji and in eight directions represented by the eight-diagrams.

It is said to have been created by Dong Haichuan (1813-1882) who was born in Wen'an County, Hebei Province, and served as a wushu master in a royal family of the Qing court - as a result of enlightenment by Taoist theory when he was travelling south of the Yangtze River. It first spread in Beijing and then found its way to other parts of the country and far abroad during the past century and more.

The exercise is characterized by light, quick footwork and body turns in wave-like movements when two persons are engaged in sparring practice, who are likened to "a dragon swimming in the sea, a sharp-eyed ape on the watch, a fierce tiger on a crouch and an eagle swooping down on its prey."

While one stands still or walks around, the head, neck and waist must be kept erect, the shoulders and elbows relaxed, the belly withdrawn, the chest naturally expanded, the hips and crotch properly positioned. All steps, whether solid or void, must be clear-cut when the feet are on or off the ground, as if they were treading over mire - with the ankles in contact when they move past each other.

While moving in a circular path, the inner foot should point straight forward and the outer foot turn inward, with the knees kept near and the crotch closely guarded. All body movements, including twists, turns, turnovers and "spirals," should be supple and circular.

There are two hand forms: the dragon's claw and the cow's tongue, and 16 kinds of hand movements: push, support, carry, thrust, block, parry, interception, smash, grasp, twist, hook, punch, seal, closure, dodge and stretch - all to be used in a flexible manner in attack and defence, in preemptive strikes and in dissolving the opponent's force. Every strike with the palm must hinge on the waist and be reinforced by body turns.

Externally, it is an exercise of the hands, eyes, body and feet and, internally, an exercise of the mind, willpower, energy, essence and vitality.

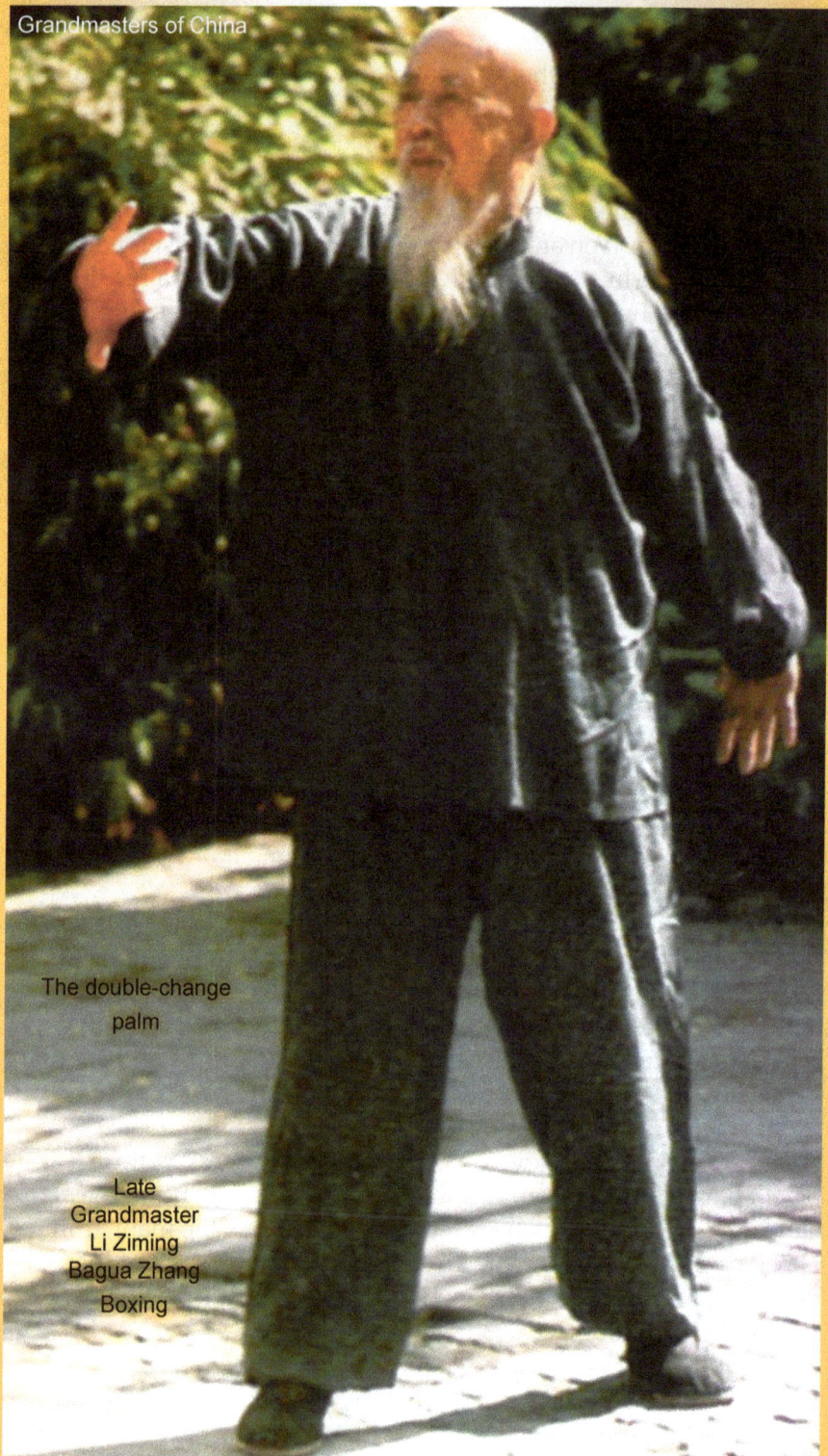

The double-change
palm

Late
Grandmaster
Li Ziming
Bagua Zhang
Boxing

The Eight-Diagram palm is practised in three phases of training: the phase of "fixed frame," the phase of "lively frame" and the phase of "changing frame".

In the first phase, all the basic movements should be done correctly with a slow tempo and a steady gait, strictly according to the requirements for every part of the body. In the second phase, all the movements should be well coordinated with a high degree of proficiency in body turns and circular walks. In the third phase, there should be harmony between the external and internal aspects, with the movements changing at one's free will and unrestricted by any fixed pattern or routine - movements "as light as a feather, as changeable as lightning and as steadfast as a rock."

There are eight palm forms, namely, the single-change palm, the double-change palm, the follow-through palm, the behind-body palm, the body turnover palm, the close-to body palm, the thrice-piercing palm and the body-turn palm, each with eight derivatives to add up to 64.

The Eight-Diagram palm may be performed by one or two persons, or in the form of free combat. According to ancient records, there are such varieties as the Arhat's Palm Exercises in 18 Circles, the Concealed Footwork in 72 Forms and the 72 Kicks, which are rarely practised today.

The exercises may also be performed with weapons like sword, broadsword and halberd, which, as the saying goes, should follow the body closely, while the body must follow the changing steps in a continuous flow of movements.

Among the short weapons used in the Eight-Diagram palm mention may be made of the double axe, the wind-and-fire wheel, the chicken's claw spear and the "judge's writing brush," which are rarely seen in other wushu schools.

As a good exercise for improving agility, speed, stamina and muscular strength, especially of the lower limbs, the Eight-Diagram Palm School has been adopted as a regular event at national wushu competitions and demonstrations.

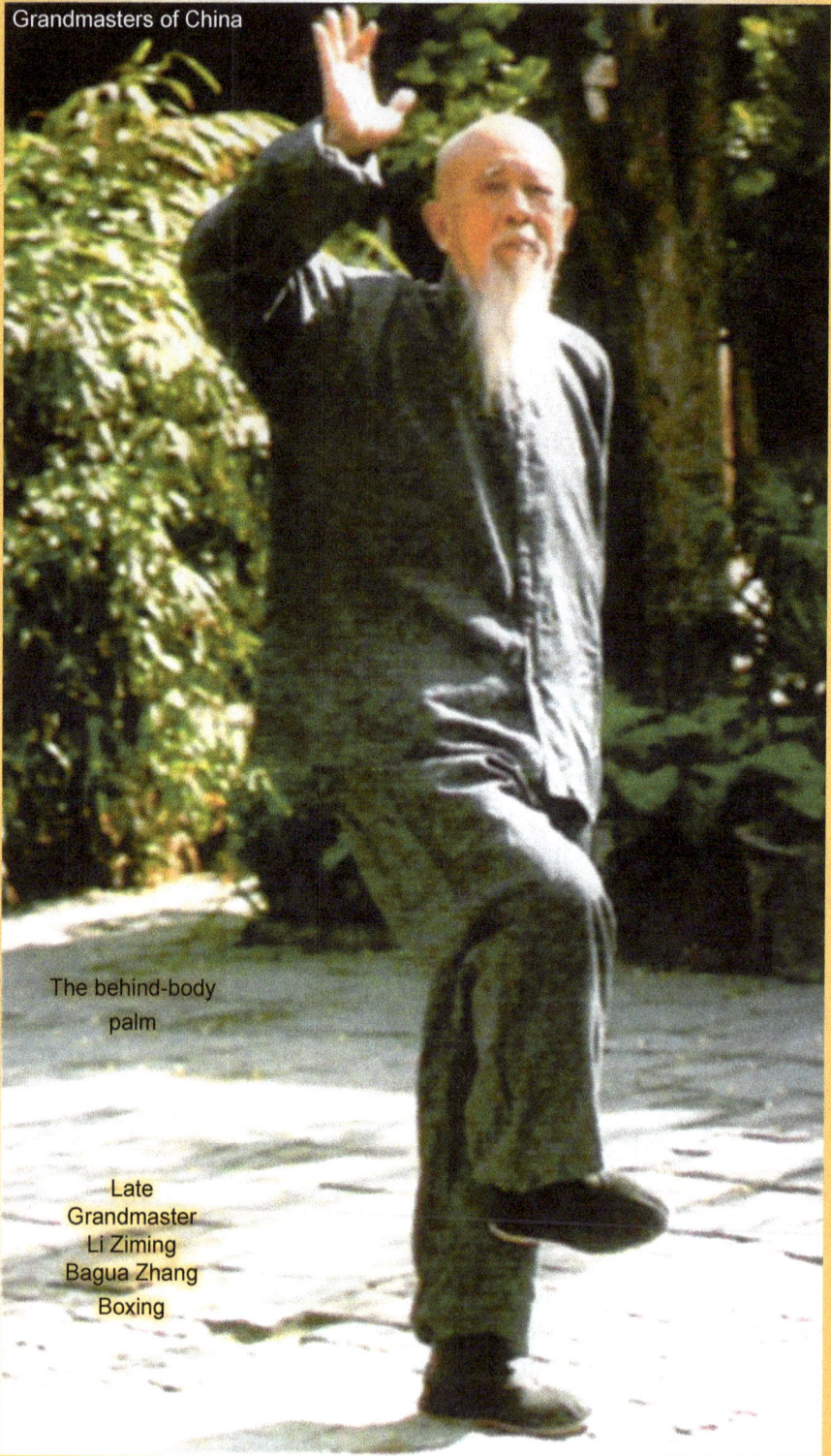

The behind-body palm

Late Grandmaster Li Ziming Bagua Zhang Boxing

Initiator of the Eight-Diagram Palm School

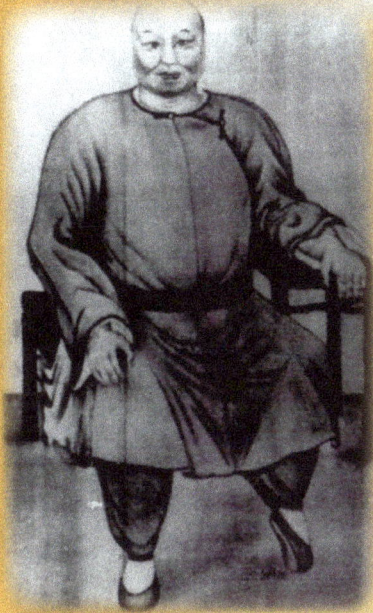

Dong Haichuan

(1798 - 1882)

Born in Wen'an County, Hebei Province, Dong Haichuan began to learn wushu in his early childhood, majoring in the "arhat boxing" of Shaolin School. Yearning to study more, he travelled widely in search of reputed masters. On Mt. Jiuhua in the southern part of Anhui Province, one of China's five sacred mountains, he saw a young Taoist practising "through the palm" exercises on a piece of slate. Out of curiosity, he proposed a bout with the boy and was defeated. After this, Dong apprenticed himself to the boy's master Bi Chengxia and stayed in the hills for several years. It was on the basis of Bi's instructions that he later evolved the Eight-Diagram palm which has enjoyed immense popularity for nearly two centuries in Beijing.

In his middle age, Dong Haichuan worked at the prince of Su's mansion, in charge of its catering office. One day a big banquet was held in the dining hall, which was so crowded that the waiters had a hard job of it serving the guests. But Dong moved easily among the tables, to the amazement of all present. He gained immediate fame for his agility and wushu skills and an endless stream of admirers implored him to teach them.

At that time Yang Luchan, founder of the Yang-style taijiquan,

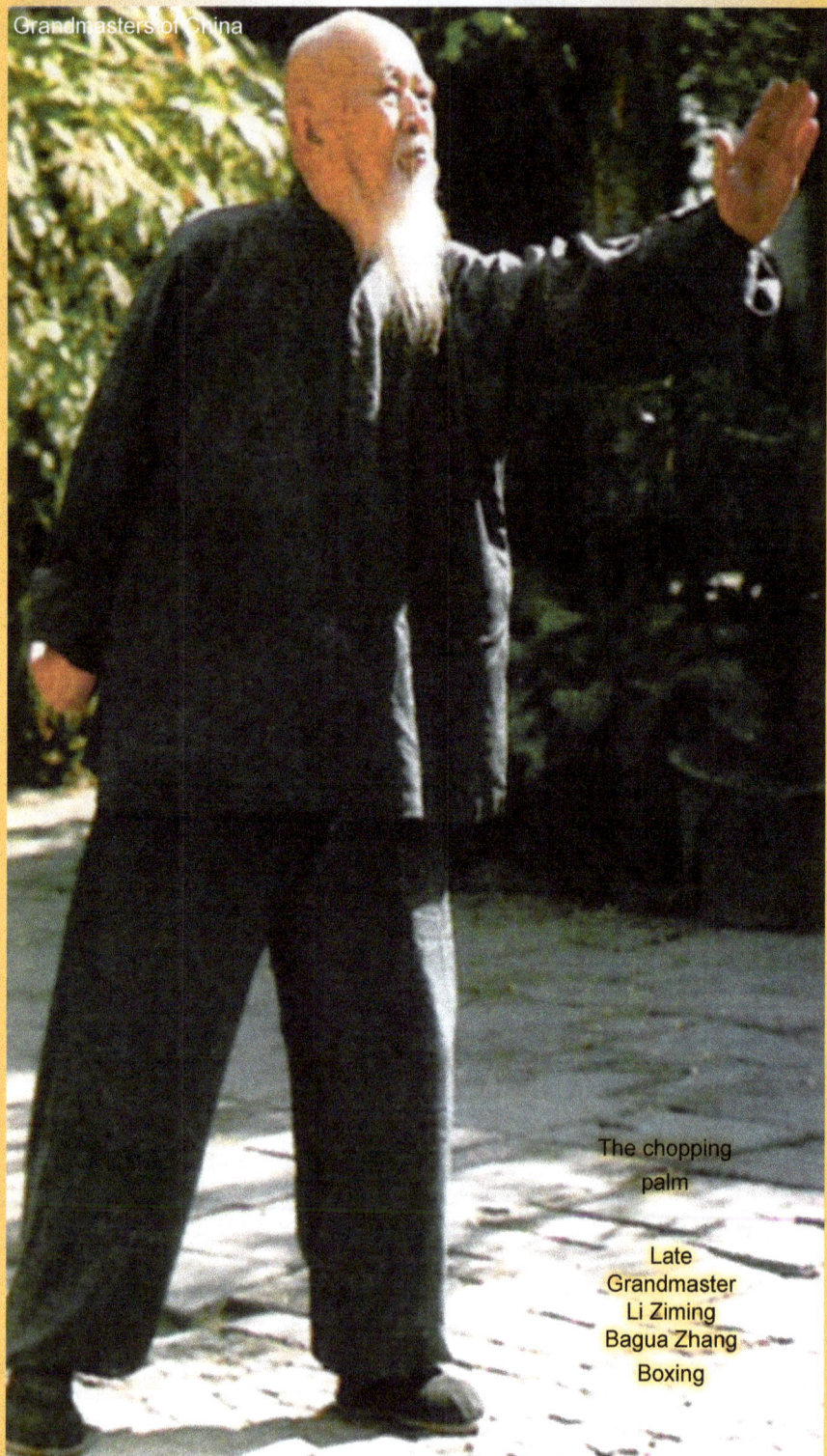

The chopping
palm

Late
Grandmaster
Li Ziming
Bagua Zhang
Boxing

was teaching wushu at the prince of Duan's mansion. A fight was arranged between him and Dong Haichuan. The three-day competition proved to be a draw and the two rivals became fast friends - an event that has gone down in wushu annals as an interesting anecdote. Later on Dong became the prince of Su's bodyguard while continuing to teach the Eight-Diagram palm in and outside his mansion.

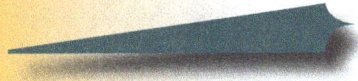

A fight was arranged between him and Dong Haichuan. The three-day competition proved to be a draw and the two rivals became fast friends...

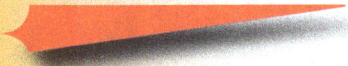

As a matter of fact, many tales have been told about Dong Haichuan's honesty, chivalry, accomplishments in martial arts and sense of justice in redressing wrongs. One night a jealous wushu master and his wife sneaked into Dong's home to kill him. No sooner had the murderer raised his spear when Dong jumped out of his bed and gave the intruders a light slap on the back, which made them kiss the ground. "Get out, you good-for-nothings without the least sense of morality as a wushu master!" Dong shouted in great anger, but he did nothing more to avenge himself.

Dong Haichuan had 72 proteges among whom Yin Fu, Song Changrong, Liu Dekuan, Cheng Tinghua, Liu Fengchu, Ma Gui, Ma Huaiqi and Zhang Zhaodong were known as the "Eight Great Disciples."

Dong Haichuan died in 1882 at the age of 84. He was buried beside the Red Bridge outside Beijing's Dongzhi Gate, with an epitaph written by his followers in praise of his glorious life. The tomb was moved to Wan'an Cemetery in 1980, at a solemn ceremony attended by hundreds of people from all walks of life.

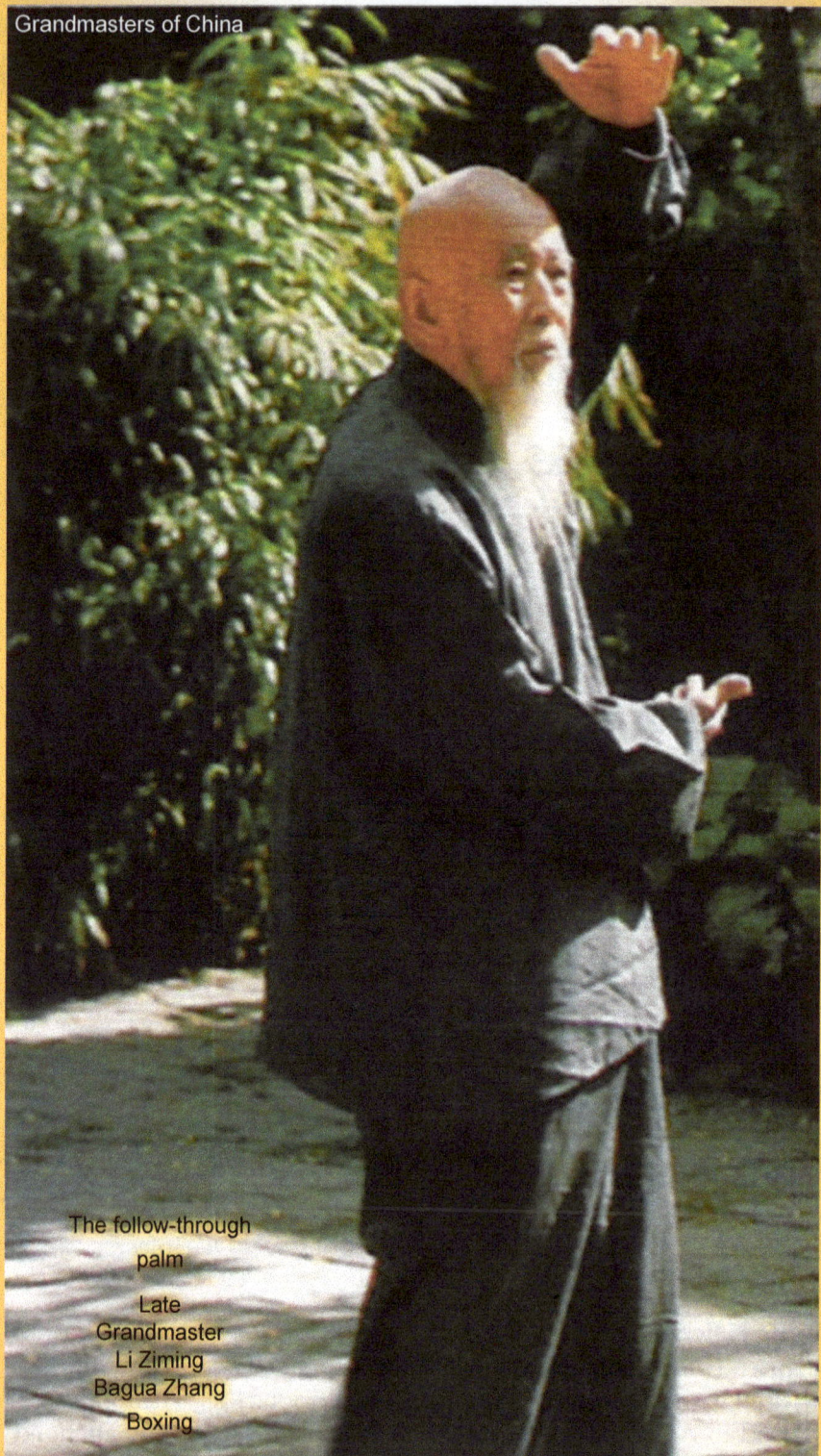

The follow-through palm

Late Grandmaster Li Ziming Bagua Zhang Boxing

Li Ziming
(1902 - 1993)

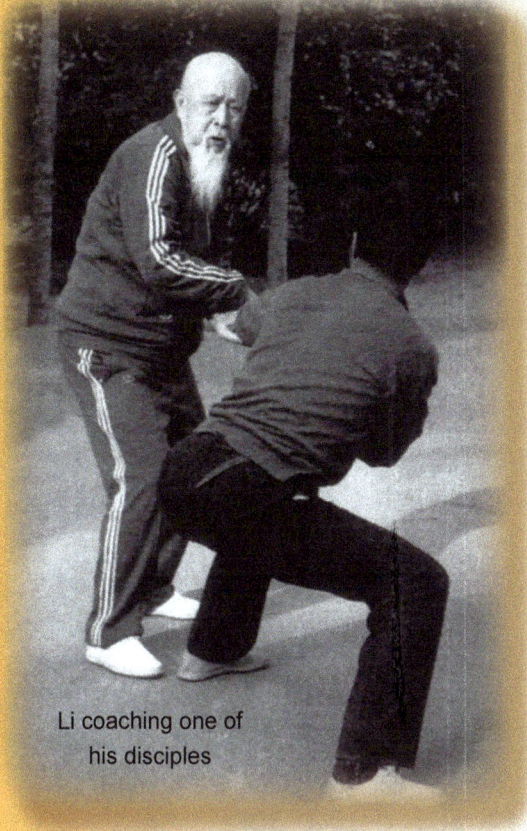

Li coaching one of his disciples

Li Ziming was born into a scholar's family in Jixian County, Hebei Province. His father, a teacher of an old-fashioned private school, wanted him to be a prominent man of letters. But almost all children in Jixian, known as "the home town of martial arts," are taught pugilism from the age of six or seven.

One day Li Ziming was surrounded by a group of urchins who called him a "pale-faced weakling." He defied them and was given a sound beating. Swallowing up his tears, the poor boy made up his mind to pick up the art of self-defence. His father brought him to his maternal uncle Si Shuchang, a reputed wushu master versed in Shaolin, Form-Will, Taiji and Bagua Zhang (Eight-Diagram Palm) exercises he had learned as a hired labourer since childhood.

Li Ziming would get up before dawn every day to practise wushu under his uncle's instruction. It was not long before his uncle died of disease. The boy was so grieved that he also fell ill. Seeing him in delicate health, Liang Zhenpu, one of his father's friends, advised him strongly to go on with wushu training as the only way to recovery. Liang had learnt Bagua Zhang from its orthodox inheritor Dong Haichuan personally when he worked as an apprentice in Beijing.

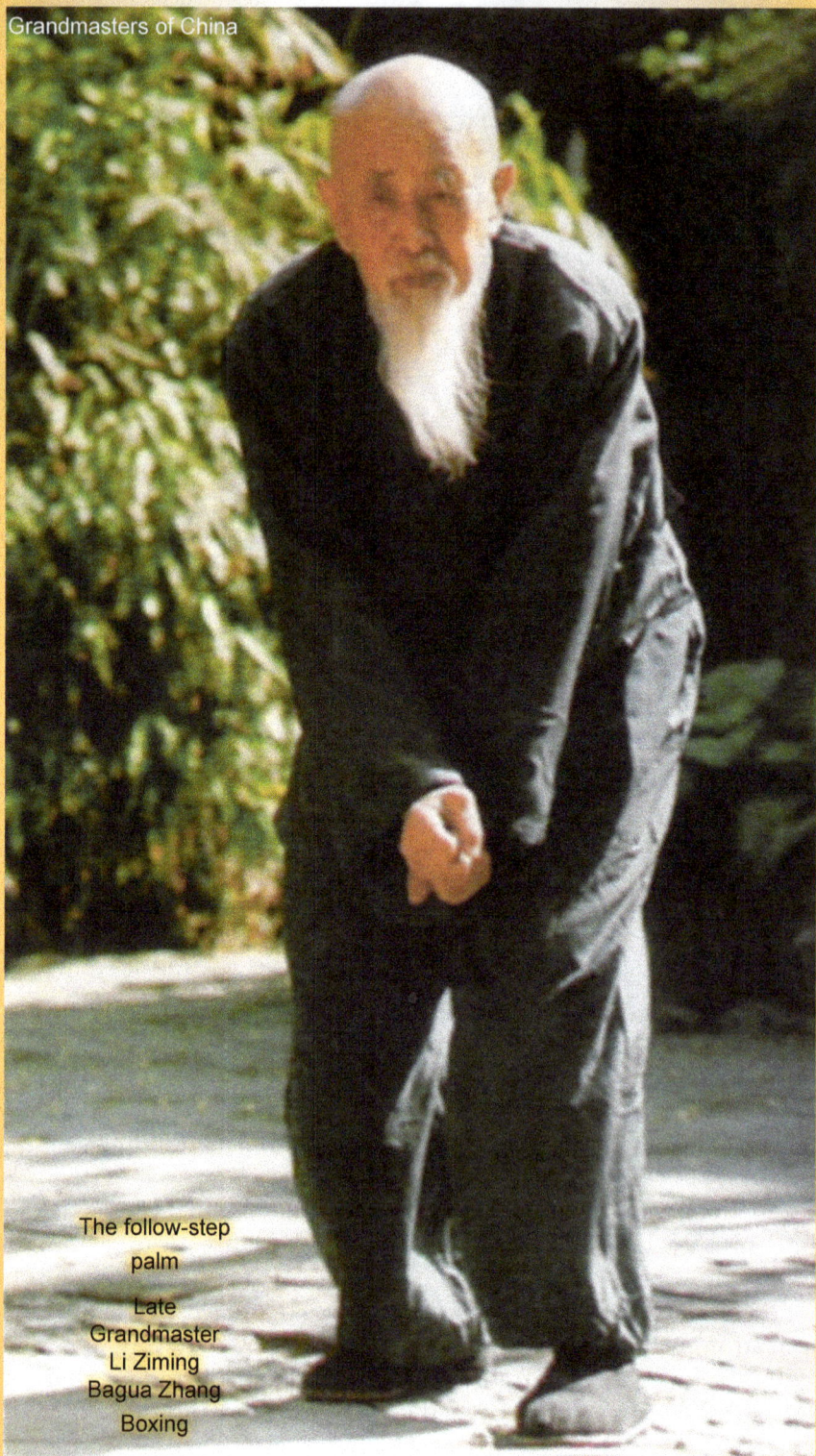

The follow-step
palm

Late
Grandmaster
Li Ziming
Bagua Zhang
Boxing

Seeing a bright boy in Li Ziming, he readily accepted him as his disciple when he returned to Jixian County.

Liang taught Li the skills of circular walk, concentrating first on the coordination between the external work of the eyes and palm and body movements on the one hand and the internal work of the mind, vitality and essence on the other, and then on the harmony among the lower, middle and upper parts of the body. Through more than ten years arduous training, Li gained a thorough comprehension of the eight-diagram palm exercises and could do every movement with great virtuosity and precision.

Many people requested Li Ziming to teach them wushu. His fame aroused jealousy in one of the villagers who had bullied Li Ziming in childhood. The bully had never stopped practising wushu while leading a vagabond life in the following years. Making nothing of that "feeble scholar," he attacked Li from behind one pitch-dark night. With a "white tiger's leap over the stream," Li turned round and gave the sneaker a "clamp with both fists on the ears," which sent him crawling on the ground. He struggled up to his feet and tried to hit Li's temple with his index and middle fingers, a traditional forte that often proved fatal. Using his "eight-diagram walk," Li circled around his opponent and evaded every attack from him. Finally, he knocked down his foe with a powerful strike of the palm. And his parting words were: "Honesty is the best policy in wushu. Always remember this and behave yourself!"

Li Ziming came to Tianjin to learn a trade at the age of 24. He was harassed by a group of ruffians at the railway station. But he beat them all. "I'm deeply sorry for the fight," he said to his friends later. "But I couldn't help it in this crazy world of ours. Bad eggs are bound to end up badly."

He came to Beijing in 1938 to earn a living at a bookstore and became an underground worker for the cause of liberation some years later. After the city was liberated in 1948, he worked as a manager of the Beijing Bean Sauce Factory, the East District Food Factory and Beijing No. 2 Food Factory until he retired in 1985. But he has not ceased to be a wushu coach. During the past decades, he has trained four generations of disciples now scattered in some 30 cities in the country and beyond it - Japan, Singapore, Norway,

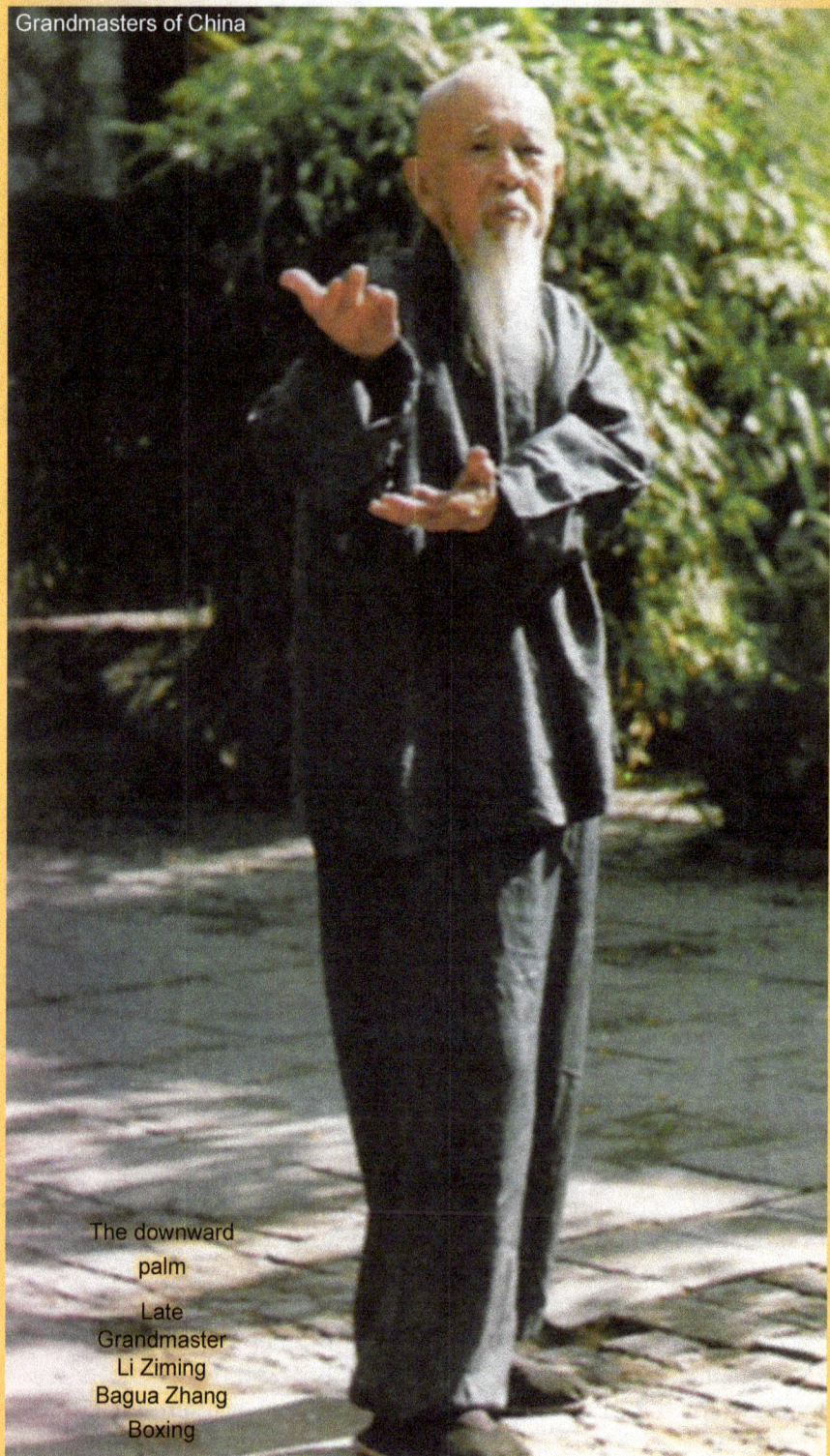

The downward
palm

Late
Grandmaster
Li Ziming
Bagua Zhang
Boxing

Austria and the
United States.

He and
his colleagues
set up 21
"eight-
diagram
palm"
coaching
stations in
Beijing. Among
their 2,000
graduates more
than a thousand
were instructed by
Li Ziming himself.

He served as
president of the
Beijing Eight-
Diagram palm
Society until his
passing, a post he
richly deserved and
enjoyed very much.

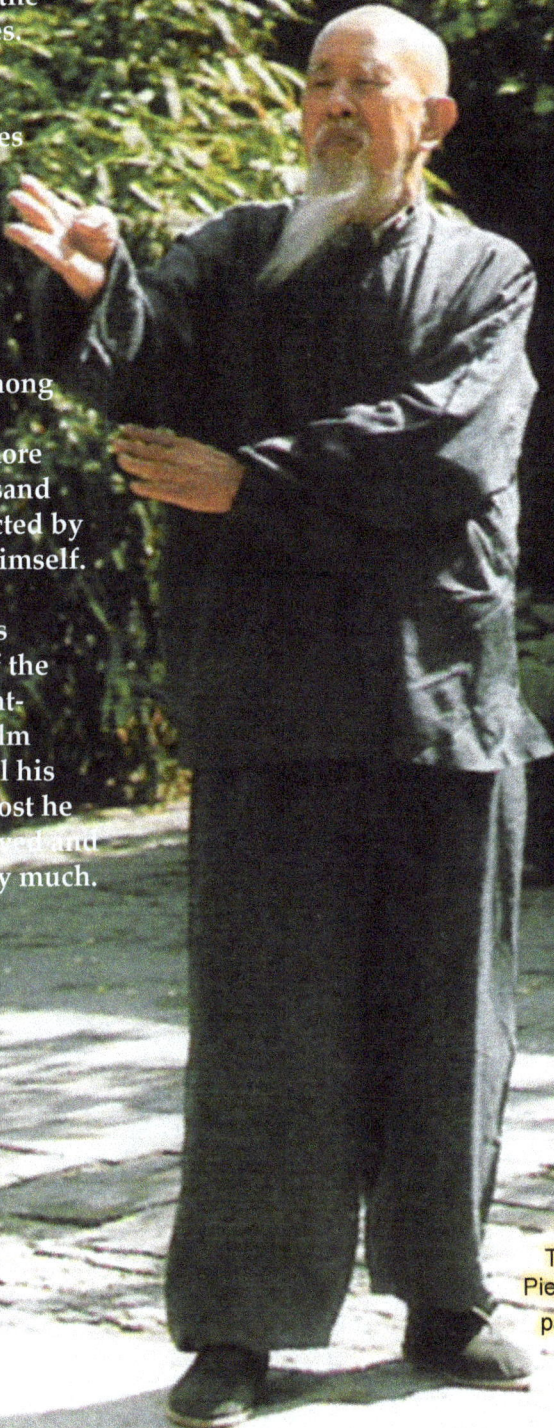

The
Piercing
palm

Grandmaster Tian Hui and his Unorthodox Bagua

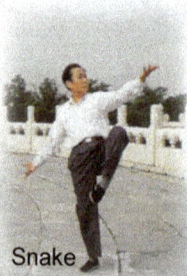

Snake

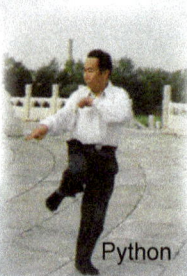

Python

Eight Separate Animal Forms: Snake, Lion, Tiger, Bear, Python, Monkey, Horse, and Eagle (Roc).

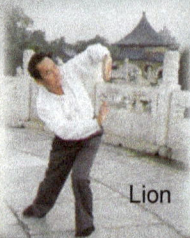

Lion

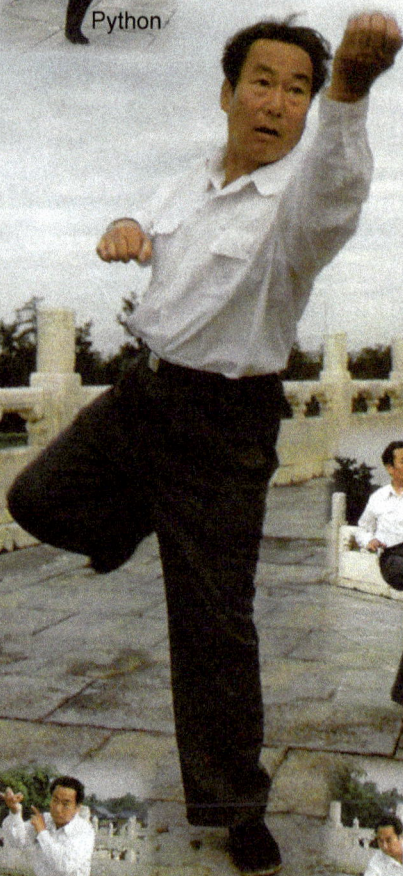

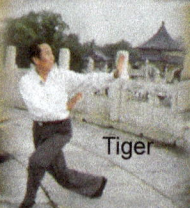

Tiger

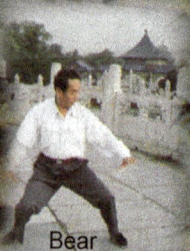

Bear

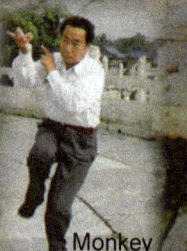

Monkey

Horse

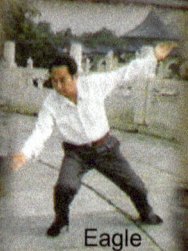

Eagle

Tian Hui emerged in the 1980s teaching wushu and writing books in Beijing. His Bagua Zhang (Eight-Diagram palm) routine is different from the orthodox one founded by Dong Haichuan; it has come down from his ancestors without being made public outside his family.

In the early 17th century, the Tians were engaged in the business of saltworks by Bohai Sea. One of the family, Tian Houjie, was just-minded and devoted to martial arts. At that time, the Ming Dynasty had just fallen and many Loyalists bore hatred to the Qing rulers of Manchu nationality and became Buddhist or Taoist monks in the hills, awaiting opportunities to overthrow the new monarchy. Tian Houjie left home and no one knew his whereabouts. Then one of his relatives, Tian Xuan, also disappeared from the family.

Many, many years later, a travel-stained Taoist came to the Tians', claiming himself to be Tian Xuan. But no one could identify him until he told many things about his childhood. They were surprised to know that he and Tian Houjie had settled down in a Taoist monastery in Emei Mountains in Sichuan Province and joined a secret anti-Qing organization. Both had learned the martial art of Bagua Zhang from two masters named Bai Yun (Purple Cloud) and Jing Yun (Quiet Cloud).

Tian Xuan had come home to pass on the fighting skills to his relatives, on promise that they would neither serve the Qing court nor teach their skills to Manchu nationals. He accepted some Tian family members as his disciples to whom he taught all the basics of Bagua Zhang before he returned to Emei Mountains. Since then this school of wushu has been handed down in the family and Tian Hui is the ninth generation of followers. Today, his son, Tian Keyan carries the style onward.

The Bagua Zhang exercises, as inherited by the Tians, consist of two routines, xiantian (congenital) and houtian (acquired). It is different from the more popular Dong Haichuan style in many respects, especially in footwork. While moving about in a circular path, the performer looks like an eagle circling in the sky rather than a person treading on mire. The system is divided into eight separate animal forms – Python, Lion, Tiger, Bear, Snake, Monkey, Horse, and Eagle.

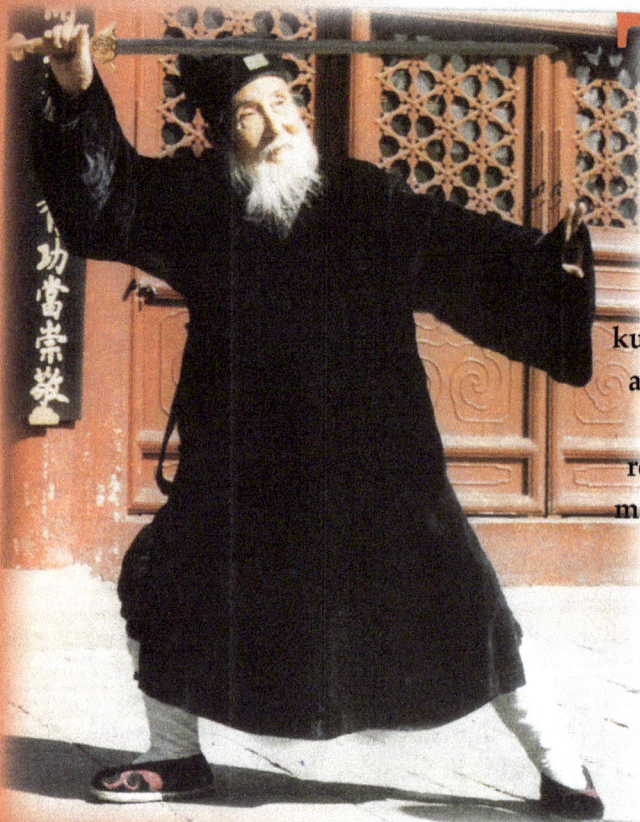

The Taoists of Baiyun (White Cloud) Temple make a point of regular kungfu practice as an indispensable part of their religious life and means of spiritual sublimation.

Top: Reverend An Shengyuan practicing taiji swordplay

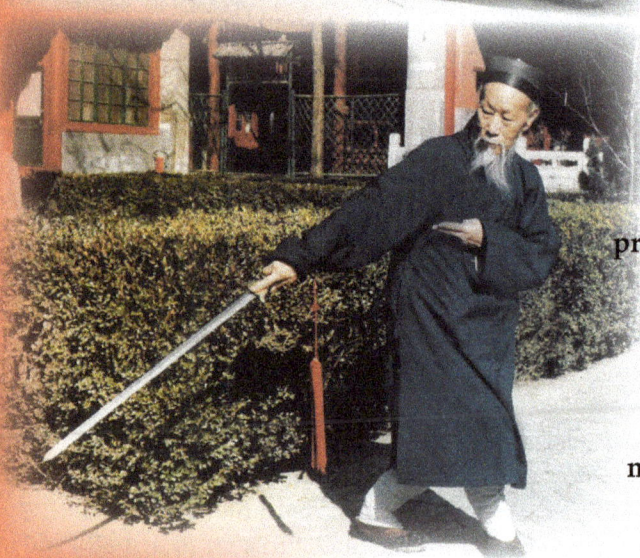

Bottom: Reverend Cai Zhenyang practicing Lu Zu's swordplay

Opposite: Rev. An plays a movement of the primeval taiji boxing

TAOIST WIZARDS OF

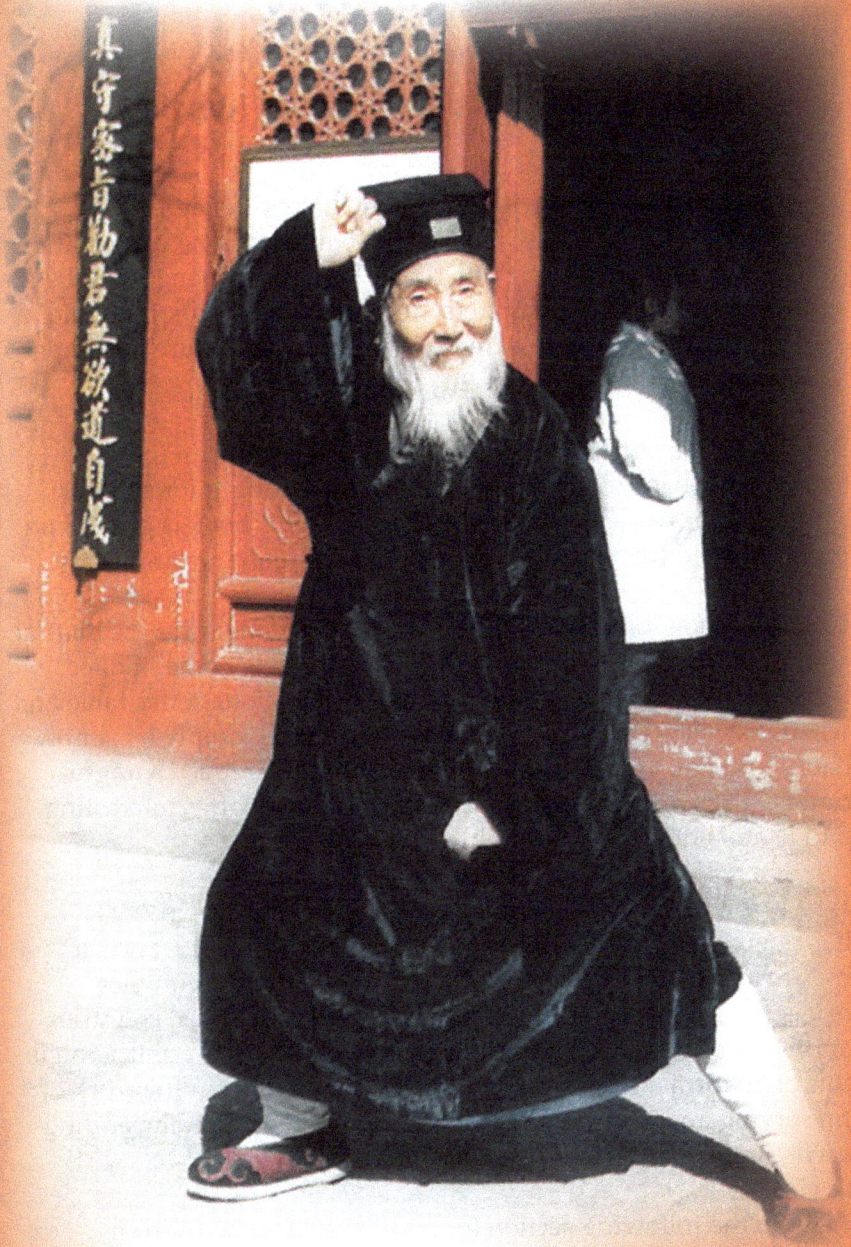

BEIJING'S
WHITE CLOUD TEMPLE

Treasures of Traditional Chinese Kungfu

This book has chronicled some who were considered "living treasures" of Chinese martial arts culture. Some were martial art creators like Dong's Bagua or Wang's Dacheng School and some were only transmitters. In both cases, their stories and teachings are truly timeless treasures from which future generations may benefit and learn.

Reprinting the original 1990 *Grandmasters* magazine in this book format has helped preserve traditional kungfu for another generation or two. Even longer perhaps, as this book is printed on premium acid free paper for an archival addition to your library.

Use your book to preserve and promote traditional Chinese martial art culture for generations of martial artists yet to come. Collect and place all the issues of *Grandmasters of China* on your coffee table and when you are asked, "What is Chinese Kungfu?", reply by simply handing them any volume of this **Traditional Chinese Kungfu Series.** Each volume of the series makes a handsome, interesting, and useful addition to your library or coffee table.

What was *Martial Arts of China* newsstand magazines in 1990 has now become this series of hardcover books in 2012, known as, *Grandmasters of China*. In total there were twelve volumes originally published as newsstand magazines in fifteen countries and Southern Mantis Press has slated them all for re-publication in this book format beginning with this issue. Join us in the work of preserving and promoting traditional Chinese Kungfu by adding each volume of this series to your library!

Refer to the following section for additional Resources from Southern Mantis Press on traditional Chinese Kungfu:

- China National Kungfu Survey Videos

- MantisFlix™ Hong Kong Survey Videos

- Additional Southern Mantis Press Publications

RESOURCES

資源

TRADITIONAL MARTIAL ARTS

OF

CHINA

AND

HONG KONG

AND

HAKKA

SOUTHERN PRAYING MANTIS

KUNGFU

CHINA NATIONAL KUNGFU SURVEY ON VIDEO

A 3 Year National Survey of China's Kung Fu by the Government!

About the Survey

Beginning 1983, the China State Sports Commission mobilized some 8,000 workers at national and local levels who travelled to the remotest corners of China to call on 15,000 old kungfu masters.

Ending in 1986, the **China National Kungfu Survey** determined there still exists some 130 different schools, each with its own distinctive origin, features and principles.

A set of books were compiled about the 130 schools with a total of 650,000 words to form a martial art encyclopedia. In addition, some 480 old manuals, 390 ancient weapons and 30 other articles, which are rare antiques with a high value for traditional wushu research, were collected.

Almost all the routines contained in the newly compiled books were recorded on video tapes with a total length of several hundred hours. The results of this National Survey have produced the most valuable asset in the history of Chinese Kungfu! Collect every hour of these rare treasures! Just as they were recorded-in their unedited version!

Details of the Survey

- Three Year National Survey of China
- 8,000 Researchers / Field Workers
- 15,000 Kungfu Masters Interviewed
- Over 400 Hours of Videotape
- All 28 Provinces Surveyed
- Direct to You - Unedited!

About the Content

Unless noted otherwise all programs are narrated in Chinese. Quality of the programs vary according to the original format. See each program description for details on content.

CHINA NATIONAL KUNGFU SURVEY ON VIDEO

A 3 Year National Survey of China's Kung Fu by the Government!

As a gem in the treasure house of China's ancient culture, martial art (wushu) has existed for thousands of years. Yet the whole picture of this form of traditional martial arts had remained unclear until the mid 1980s, when enormous work was done to excavate the ancient routines and weapons across the country, culminating in an exhibition that was held in Beijing's Palace Museum in March 1986.

From the middle of 1983, the Physical Culture and Sports Commissions and Wushu Associations at national and local levels mobilized some 8,000 people in the research work. Travelling to the remotest corners of our vast China, they called on 15,000 old wushu masters. The project cost about one million yuan and had no parallel in China's history of sports.

130 Branches

Although many attempts had been made in the past to determine the number of branches or schools of wushu, no definite answer could be obtained and materials collected were far from complete or systematic. Now, as a result of the China National Kungfu Survey, we can tell that there are some 130 different schools, each with an origin, style, special features and principles that it may call its own.

Some schools on the verge of extinction have come to light. Yuejiaquan, for instance, was confirmed to have been evolved by Yue Fei (1103-1142), a famous general in the Song Dynasty, and carried on by his descendants living in seclusion in Hubei Province since he was murdered by treacherous court officials. Other wushu schools saved from extinction include Tianzhi Siquan in Gansu and Zangquan (Tibetan boxing) in Qinghai in northwestern China, and Chuanquan (boxing on boats) in the coastal province of Zhejiang.

A clearer picture has been made of the various wushu forms popular among the ethnic groups living in the southern and southwestern parts of the country. It was on the basis of these extensive investigations that a whole set of books were compiled about the wushu schools

CHINA NATIONAL KUNGFU SURVEY ON VIDEO

A 3 Year National Survey of China's Kung Fu by the Government!

with a total of 650,000 words to form an encyclopaedia of wushu with detailed information on the skills, history and geographical distribution of all schools and exercises, barehanded or with weapons.

Three Contributions

To collect materials scattered widely among the folk, the survey initiated a "three contribution campaign" - contribution of wushu manuals, ancient weapons and technical expertise - offering Lion Prizes for the donors. This awakened patriotic enthusiasm among those possessed of what the State wanted to collect.

The State Physical Culture and Sports Commission alone received 480 manuals, 390 ancient weapons and 30 other articles which are mostly rare antiques or have a high value for research. Among the manuals awarded first prizes are hand copies of *ABCs of Swordplay*, *On Cudgelplay, Tongbeiquan in 108 Forms*, and *Diagrams of the Single Scimitar Exercise* copied in 1715 and *Xingyiquan (Form-and-Will Boxing)* copied in the last century - all with lucid instructions and annotations.

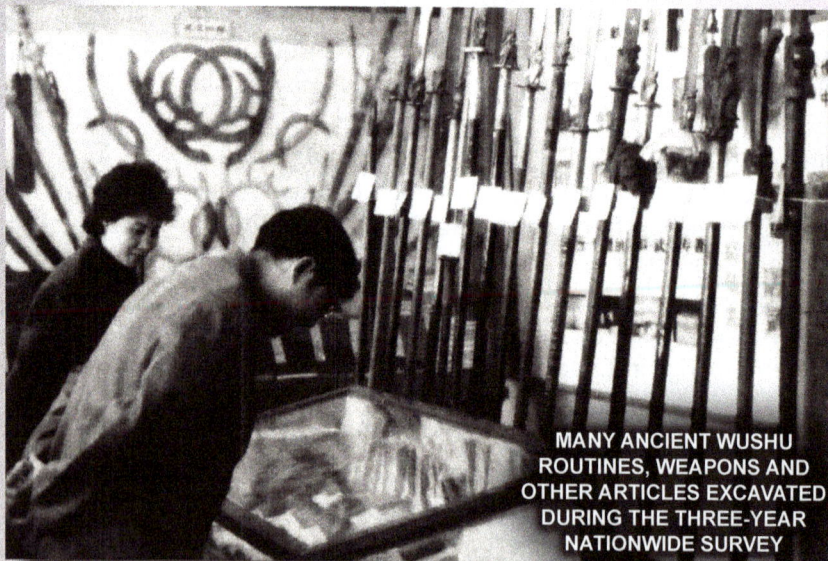

MANY ANCIENT WUSHU ROUTINES, WEAPONS AND OTHER ARTICLES EXCAVATED DURING THE THREE-YEAR NATIONWIDE SURVEY

CHINA NATIONAL KUNGFU SURVEY ON VIDEO

A 3 Year National Survey of China's Kung Fu by the Government!

The weaponry includes a dagger-axe made in Sichuan during the Period of Warring States (475-221 BC), a sword with a ring handle made during the Tang Dynasty (618-907), an iron whip during the Yuan Dynasty (1271-1368), and General's Scimitar and a cudgel during the Ming Dynasty (1368-1644), as well as some wushu weapons used by well-known historical figures.

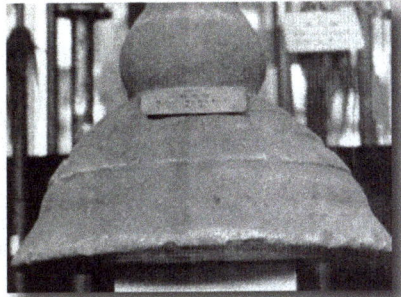

The stone sandals and headgear (stone cap - photo right), iron broadswords and a strength-exercise frame on display at the exhibition were evidently used in ancient times for training purposes. An armour unearthed in Zhejiang Province is said to have been worn by a martial hero in the Qing Dynasty (1644-1911). There was a photograph taken in Zhejiang in 1928 of the applicants for a state examination in martial arts, and a banner presented to a wushu group in Fujian Province during its visit to Southeast Asia in 1929 - the first ever sent abroad according to recent studies.

A Lever for Scientific Research

Down through the ages wushu routines have been handed down chiefly through demonstrations and by word of mouth. Stored up only in the minds of aging masters, many are in imminent danger of dying out. It was in view of this that almost all the routines contained in the compiled books were recorded on video tapes with a total length worth some 400 hours. In one of the cassettes were recorded performances given by two wushu masters in their eighties in Hunan Province who passed away shortly afterwards. We cannot but treasure all the records taken in the course of the China National Kungfu Survey as perhaps the most valuable asset in the history of Chinese Kungfu!

Today more and more people have come to realize that wushu should be studied in the light of modern science, inasmuch as it is

97

CHINA NATIONAL KUNGFU SURVEY ON VIDEO

A 3 Year National Survey of China's Kung Fu by the Government!

closely associated with physiology of exercise, sports medicine, biomechanics, psychology, ethics, aesthetics, history, etc. We are glad that this Survey has served as a lever for scientific research.

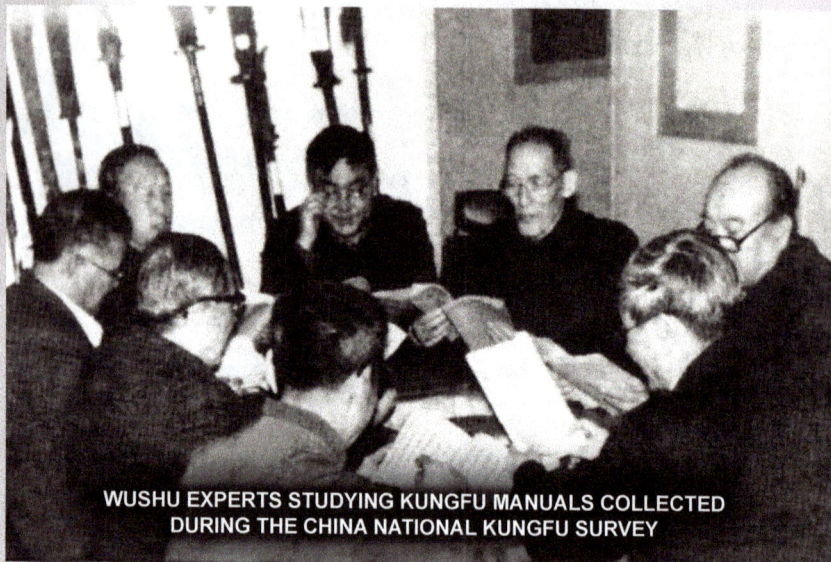

WUSHU EXPERTS STUDYING KUNGFU MANUALS COLLECTED DURING THE CHINA NATIONAL KUNGFU SURVEY

START YOUR SURVEY VIDEO COLLECTION TODAY!

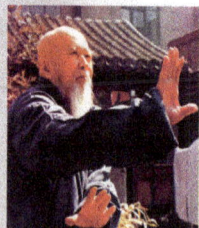

Survey 103: Wushu, Shaolin, Tai Chi Highlights
Short briefs on dozens of wushu styles; men and women at their wushu best: Changquan; Taijiquan; Nanquan; Broadsword; Double edge sword; staff; spear; Hsing I Chuan; Baguazhang; Tongbelquan; Fanziquan; Ditangquan; North Mantis boxing; Snake boxing; Eagle boxing; Drunken boxing; Monkey boxing; Drunken sword boxing; Monkey staff; Baguazhang broadsword; double straight sword; double daggers; double broadswords; double hook swords; 3 section staff; double whip chains; rope dart; broadsword and whip chain; paired fighting; 3 man fight routine; spear vs. double broadsword; double spear

CHINA NATIONAL KUNGFU SURVEY ON VIDEO

A 3 Year National Survey of China's Kung Fu by the Government!

vs. broadsword; open hand vs. broadsword and staff; group performance; followed by Shaolin temple footage; Shaolin boxers; Shaolin relics; Luohanquan; Wuzhongquan; Changquan (Yu Shaowen); Shaolin staff, broadsword; Ditang; Chainwhip; Nan Shaolin; 3 man fighting; Li Lianjie's childhood training and family; Wu Bin; group training; Chen Xaiowang; Yang Zhenduo; Sun Taichi (Sun Jinyu); Wu Tai Chi (Wu Yinhua); Feng Zhiqiang; group training; and much more! 60 min. Chinese. **KFS103**

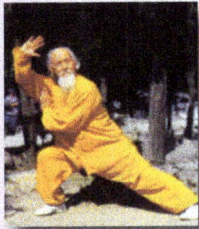

Survey 104: Emei and Wudang Boxing

Emei Mountain temples; swords; open hand forms; 2 man form; Hoquan; Snake; Daggers; 9 section whip; Spear vs. broadsword; Luohan boxing; Spade; Spear; 3 section staff; Shandong—Double axes; open hand form; Dragon hooks; Tonfas; Double wheels; Double hooks; 9 section whip and broadsword; Rake vs. staff; Wudang Mountain—Sword; Li Xia's Jian; Tongbei; 8 Immortals Drunken sword; Paired fighting; Duck boxing; White Crane; Dog boxing; Mantis boxing; Monkey vs. Drunken; Eagle; Eagle vs. Snake; Yue Fie's Temple Hangzhou West Lake; Hsing I; 2 man Hsing I; Baguazhang; Dong Hai Chuan's grave; Li Ziming; Bagua demo; Baguazhang Broadsword; Bagua pushhands; Hou Shuying (Wonders of Qigong) Hard Qigong; Performance Wushu; staff; Li Xia spear; Paired fighting; Drunken style vs. Changquan; Shorinji Kenpo; staff vs. 3 section staff; open hand vs. broadsword & spear; broadsword & shield vs. staff & open hand; 3 man fighting. 60 min. Chinese Language. **KFS104**

Survey 108: "A Collection of Chinese Kungfu"

A good documentary to introduce the wonders of Chinese kungfu!; Inspire anyone to take up training!; Beautiful Hanzhou West Lake; group performances; Feng Quiying spear; Sledgehammer vs. staff; staff; double broadsword; double hook swords; Eagle; Snake; 3 man fight routines; Sanda free sparring; weapons; training; staff; double broadsword; Emei double daggers; Fanziquan; Ditangquan; 3 section staff vs. staff; Zuiquan; Ying Qigong (Hard Qigong); Taijiquan sword; Tongbeiquan; 3 section staff; sword; Ying Qigong; 78 yr old and his 100 lb Kwandao; Ying Qigong; Nanquan; 9 section whip chain; double sword; 2 man Chinna; North Mantis; Kwandao;

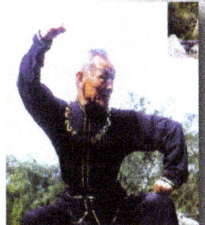

CHINA NATIONAL KUNGFU SURVEY ON VIDEO

A 3 Year National Survey of China's Kung Fu by the Government!

Survey 108 Con't

Ying Qigong; Broadsword; Zuijien; Nanquan; 2 man routine; broadsword; staff; broadsword/shield vs. 3 section staff; broadsword and 9 section whip chain; Snake boxing vs. Eagle boxing; Ying Qigong (man supports 4000 lbs on abdomen). 49 min. Chinese Language. **KFS108**

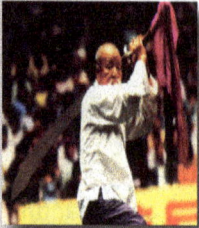

Survey 113: Kungfu Physical Festival

1,000 Nanquan performers!; Temple of Heaven; Taiji demo; Master Li's Dragon broadsword; two hand sword; Nanquan; staff; sword; history of wushu; Xian Terracotta soldiers; ancient books; Monkey King; Taiji; Shaolin; Drunken; Chen's Village; Chen's push hands; group Taiji; Shaolln Temple; Shaolin form; paired fighting; Temples; Wudang Temple; Chen's group Taiji; Yang Zhenduo; Chen Xiaowang; Feng Zhi Qiang; children's broadsword; Drunken sword; Kwandao; Monkey staff; broadsword vs. 9 section whip; broadsword; Double Dragon hooks; Double Tonfa; Double circle wheels; paired fighting group performance; auditorium performance; Bagua Zhang; Eagle; Northern Mantis; Crane; Monkey; Opera; Li Lianjie; IWF; Xucai; Competition sword; staff; Great Wall; broadsword; Taiji; Longfist Changquan; Southfist Nanquan; Free style sparring; childrens paired fighting; President Nixon; Henry Kisslnger; Japanese styles; Bagua Zhang; Shorinji Kenpo; USA Team; Master Zhang Wenguang; competitions; 1,000 performers; foreign performers; large dragon dancing; forging weapons. 40 min. Chinese Language. **KFS113**

Survey 134: Old Master's Forms Survey

An outstanding collection of many old masters performing their traditional forms; 99 yr old Dragon Lin Zhiqing's double swords; 86 yr old Sha Guozheng's Baguazhang; an excellent sword routine; Feng Zhiqiang's Chen Style Taiji broadsword; 82 yr old Zhao Ziqui's Emei Huaquan; 82 yr old Ma Zhenwu's Luohan broadsword; Elder Sifu's 100 lb Kwandao; Hsing I Chuan; Baguazhang; Chaquan; Chen's Taiji; Fujowpai Tiger Claw; 5 routines of Ho gun Monkey Staff; 6 routines of Zuiquan Jian Drunken sword; 2 routines of Kwandao Play; Long Tassle Jian sword; Chen's Taiji sword; 6 routines of red tassled spear play. 60 min. Chinese Language. **KFS134**

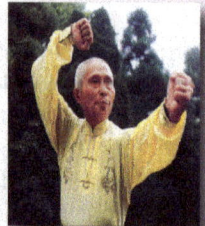

CHINA NATIONAL KUNGFU SURVEY ON VIDEO

A 3 Year National Survey of China's Kung Fu by the Government!

Survey 142: Shanxi Province Traditional Kungfu

Qinglong Claw; glitch; Nanquan; Staff; Tigerfork; Chelongquan; 6 yr old; Choy Li Fut; Chin Pin Jian; 2 man Bajiquan; 80 yr old Bench boxing; 80 yr old Nan Danquan; Hakka Nanquan; Fuzhao Eagle Nanquan; Long axe; Snake quan; Monkey quan; Northern Mantis fist; Crane boxing; Chaquan; Mizongquan; Shaolin Pao Chui; North Spring boxing; Fanziquan; Taiji group; group discussion; 9 demonstrations of Shanxi Hsing I Chuan; 82 yr old 12 Animal Hsing I; 5 Element 12 Animal Hsing I Chuan 76 yr old; 71 yr old 8 form Hsing I; 2 man Hsing I; Secret Hsing I (8 yrs old); 3 demos Hsing I; Hsing I dagger; Hsing I double needles; Hsing I wand; Museum; 4 forms of Shanxl Tongbel quan; Tongbei Yinyang Tui; 5 demonstntions of short staff; 4 demos of Gongliquan; 3 demos of 2 man Gongliquan form; Spear; Yang Zhenduo; Hslng I; Baguazhang; 84 yr old Shaolin; Longxlngquan; large straight broadsword; Shaolin Nei jia quan; Dafonshou; Double Tonfa; Tongbiquan; Rope weapon; Tongbei; Shanxi Village. 48min. Chinese Language. **KFS142**

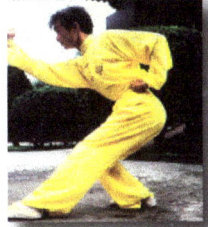

Survey 143: Complete Cha Boxing 10 Forms; Shandong Survey

Dozens of forms!; and the complete Cha Quan system. Wen Sheng Quan; Chen's Taijiquan (Pao Chui form); Shr San jian (double edge sword); Yuen Qing Quan; short staff; North Mantis; Sun Bing Quan; Si Tong quan; Dan Bin Gong; Da Hongquan; Huaquan; Ba Kwei Shou; Big Crescent Knife; Ba Zhou; Wu Zong Yi; Monk's Spade; Double hand sword; Complete Cha Quan open hand system - forms 1 through 10. 52 min. Chinese Language. **KFS143**

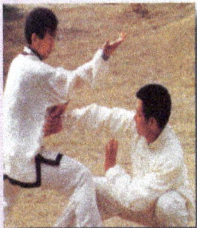

START YOUR SURVEY VIDEO COLLECTION TODAY! MORE THAN 100 HOURS OF TRADITIONAL CHINESE KUNGFU DIRECT FROM CHINA!

Email for Your Free Video Download and Complete Survey List!

info@SouthernMantisPress.com

Vol 1: Pingshan Mantis Celebration Hardcover or eBook

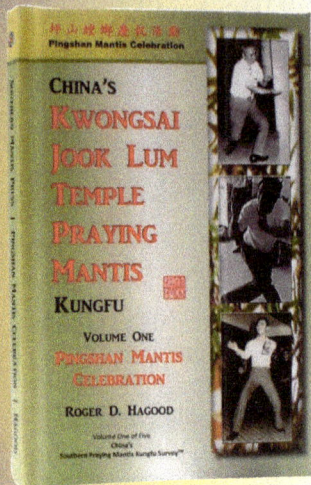

Pingshan Mantis Celebration
A rare book of China's Kwongsai Jook Lum Temple Praying Mantis Kungfu and Unicorn Culture.

Included are: Origins, history and practices of China's Kwongsai Mantis, rare and exclusive historical photographs never published before, the hometown of Kwongsai Mantis-Pingshan Town, how Wong Yuk Kong came to learn Hakka Mantis, why Wong Sifu went "mad" after a spell was cast, why Hakka Mantis is divided into "three orders" and what they are, three Wong Brothers who inherited Kwongsai Mantis, what Kwongsai Mantis boxing was taught early on and now, what happened when Kwongsai Mantis and Chu Gar first met, Hakka Mantis descending the mountain on horseback in 1917, English and Chinese translation of how Master Chung blossomed Hakka Mantis in South China, Hakka Culture along the East River, extensive interviews with inheritor Wong Yu Hua about sensitive topics, rules and regulations of Wong Yuk Kong's Mantis School, a Hakka Feast in

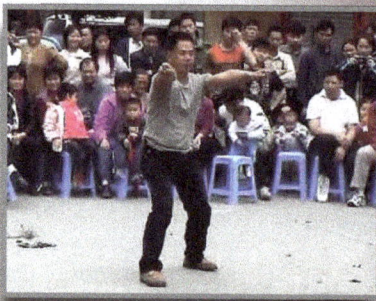

Pingshan Town, valuable Hakka Mantis resources online and off, Hakka Mantis boxing maxims and proverbs, dozens of Kwongsai Mantis boxing postures, staff, and sword pictures, rare never before published Jook Lum Mantis reliquary photographs, the Bamboo Forest Temple true heritage Dit Da liniment prescription and more.

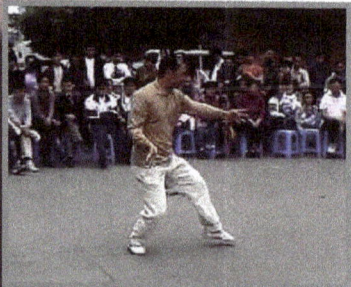

Available at Amazon, Barnes and Noble, and other fine booksellers!
Search Keywords - Southern Mantis Press

Hardcover Collector's Edition Book

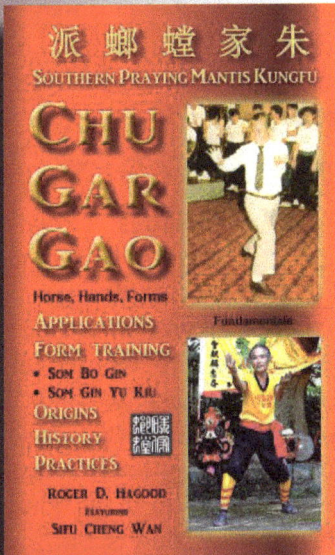

Chu Gar Gao: Southern Mantis

A rare treatise of Hakka Chu Gar Southern Praying Mantis boxing that includes: Chu Gar Mantis history, boxing transmission, six Chu Gar areas, three kinds of Chu Gar in China; Chu Gar Mantis personal records --- Sifu Chen Ching Hong, Sifu Yip Sui, Sifu Cheng Wan, Sifu Cheng Chiu, Sifu Dong Yat Long, Sifu Ma Jiuhua, Past Masters in Charge; Chu Gar applications --- Single Bridge Tsai Sao, Double Bridge Dui Jong, Mang Dan Sao Dui Jong, Ying Sao Shadow Hand, Gow Choy Hammer Fist, Locking Hands, Bridge, Tan Sao, and Ginger Fist, Double Bridge Gwak Sao, Sticky Hand and Intercepting Hand Bao Zhang Palms; Chu Gar shadowboxing forms in pictorial--Som Bo Gin (Three Step Arrow) and Som Gin Yu Kiu (Three Arrows Shaking Bridge form); and more.

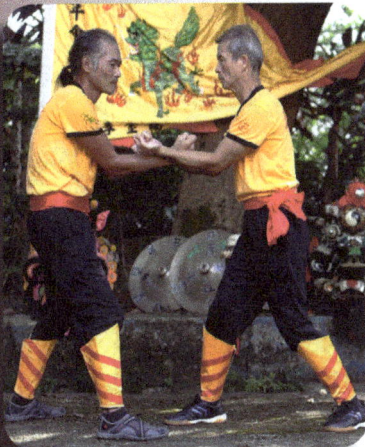

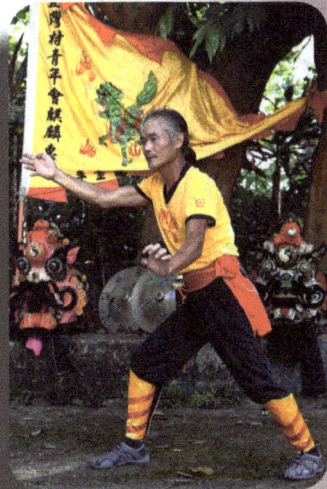

Available at Amazon, Barnes and Noble, and other fine booksellers!
Search Keywords - Southern Mantis Press

VOL 2, 3, 4: China Mantis Survey Hardcover or eBook

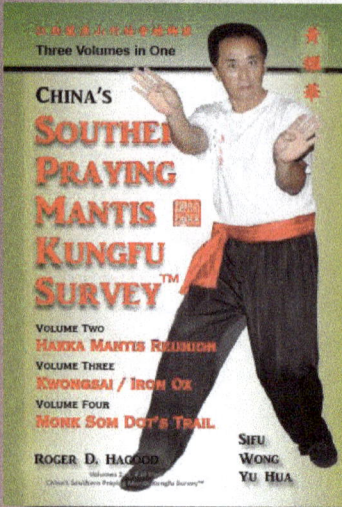

A rare three volume book of China's Hakka Kwongsai Jook Lum Temple and Iron Ox Praying Mantis boxing.

Volume Two, China Hakka Mantis Reunion, includes: Three Orders of Som Dot's Shaolin Mantis revisited, Hakka Mantis blossoms in Huizhou, Elder Lok Wei Ping a Chu Gar and Kwongsai Sifu, Chung Yel Chong teaches one form, Kwongsai and Chu Gar clash in the 40s, Sifu Wong Gok Hong takes the lion head away, Lau Say Kay Sifu plays non-standard Kwongsai Mantis, Sifu

Lai Wei Keung first Instructor in 1948, One Kwongsai form orginally taught, Two methods of beggar hands, Sifu Cho Gum, Sifu Wong Yu Hua, Fairy hands cause a slap on the rear, Lok Sifu plays 34 Plum Blossom Staff, All Mantis is one family, Lai Sifu plays 34 Plum Blossom staff and more!

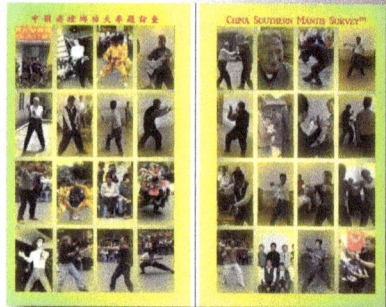

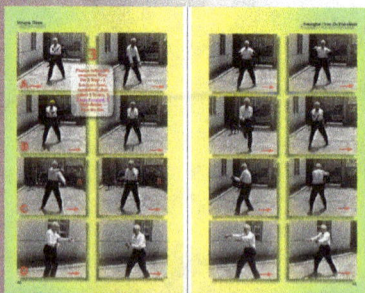

Volume Three, Kwongsai / Iron Ox Interviews, includes: Records of the elders and knowledge lost, Sifu Yao Kam Fat, Wong Yuk Kong opens Kwongsai Mantis in Hong Kong, Wong Yuk Kong visits Lao Sui's Chu Gar school, Wong Yuk Kong defeats 10 assailants, Yao Sifu plays three steps-three scissors old form, Similarities in Hakka Mantis, Yao Sifu plays 34 Plum Blossom staff, Spirit Shrine of Wong Yuk Kong, Elder Sifu Chung

VOL 2, 3, 4: Three Volumes in One Hardcover Book

Wu Xing first disciple of Chung Yel Chong, Iron Uncle Chung friend of Lam Sang, Iron Uncle Chung smokes opium with Lam Sang and Master Chung in the 1930s, Sifu Yang Gun Ming student of Chung Yel Chong, Dit Da Doctors by lineage, Hakka Mantis prohibited in the Cultural Revolution, Sifu Xu Men Fei Iron Ox Hakka Mantis, Iron Ox taught only 2 months a year, Xu Sifu plays Iron Ox Second Door form-Red Flag Staff-and Third Door form, Iron Ox challenges Wong Yuk Kong's Kwongsai Mantis, Iron Ox Secret Drill Hand not taught, and more.

Note: The hardcover book has supplemental information not contained in the eBook.

Volume Four, On Monk Som Dot's Trail / Chung Yel Chong Family Interviews, includes: Sifu Chung Wei Fei grandson of Master Chung, Master Chung Yel Chong as a boy accepted by Monk Lee, Chung Go Wah son of third ancestor Master Chung, Master Chung's boxing and Dit Da Medicine books, Third Ancestor Chung teaches Kwongsai Mantis in Hong Kong 1920s, Master Chung kills a man in self-defense, Master Chung's three generations under one roof, Sifu Lee Kok Leung outlines his Kwongsai Mantis teaching, Sifu Patrick Lee plays Mantis in Pingshan Town, Lee Sifu's History of Kwongsai Mantis, On Som Dot's Trail - Shanxi Jook Lum Temple, Oldest of the Temple Halls, Chung and Monk Lee return South six months on horseback, Kwongsai Dragon Tiger Mountain of Shaolin boxing and spiritualism, The bottom line about Kwongsai Jook Lum Temple, Lam Sang's Kwongsai spiritualism and amulet, Monk Lee Siem looks like a ghost, Jook Lum Temple in Hong Kong, Jook Lum Temple in Macau, Map of Jook Lum Temples in China with Hakka Mantis boxing, Abridged China Hakka Mantis history, Guang Wu Tang Martial Hall of Wong Yuk Kong in 2012, Mission statement of Guang Wu Tang Kwongsai Mantis, Sifu Wong Yu Hua in 2012, Miscellanies, Resources, Train in China. Kwongsai Mantis and Iron Ox boxing and staff forms in sequence, and more.

Hardcover, full color, 330+ photographs. 128 pages.

**Available at Amazon, Barnes and Noble, and other fine booksellers!
Search Keywords - Southern Mantis Press**

Hardcover Collector's Edition Book

Eighteen Buddha Hands
Kwongsai Jook Lum Temple Mantis

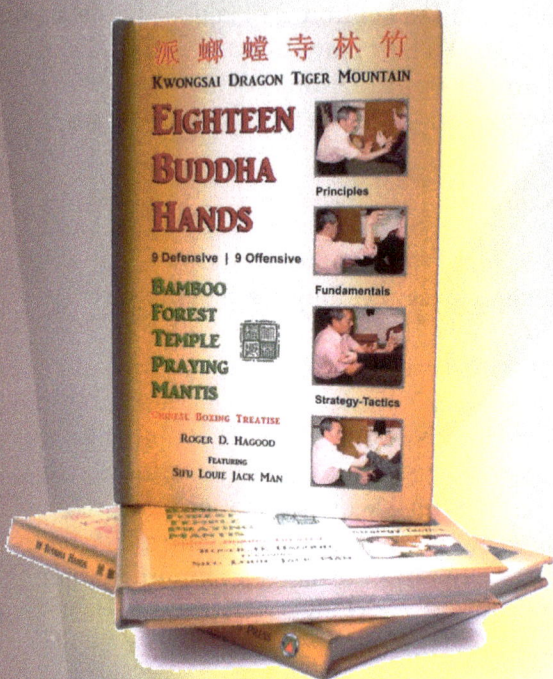

A rare instructional treatise of Chinese boxing from the Kwongsai Dragon-Tiger Mountain, Bamboo Forest Temple, Praying Mantis Clan, as transmitted by the late Grandmaster Lam Sang.

Details include stories of Lam Sang's supernatural ability such as Poison Snake Staff, Sun Gazing, and Light Body Skills. Boxing principles elaborated are Body posture, Rooting, Sinking, Center-line, Spiral power, Contact-control-strike, Intercepting and sticky hand, Bridging, Anticipating-telegraphing, Dead and live power, Form and function, 4 word secret, Dim Mak vital points and more.

Boxing Fundamentals included are Footwork: Chop, Circle, Advance, Shuffle step, Turnarounds, Side to side; Kicks, Sweeps, Takedowns, Grappling, Chin Na Seizing, Hook hands, Elbow strokes, Dui Jong, Sticky hands, Forms, and Phases of training. Eighteen Buddha Hand techniques, 9 defensive, 9 offensive, are illustrated in color with instruction in attributes, function and vital point targeting. Boxing maxims of strategy and tactics are included.

Available at Amazon, Barnes and Noble, and other fine booksellers!
Search Keywords - Southern Mantis Press

Hardcover Book: Som Bo Gin Two Man Form

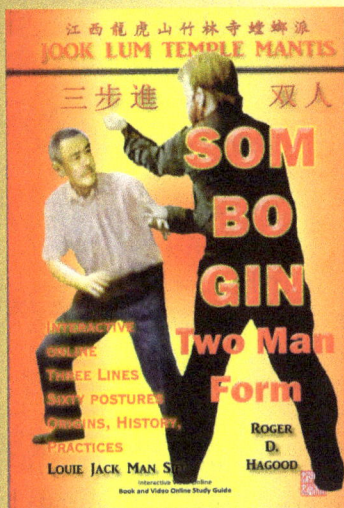

An interactive instructional treatise teaching 60 postures of the Som Bo Gin (Three Steps Forward) Two Man boxing routine of Lam Sang's Kwongsai Jook Lum Temple Praying Mantis Kungfu.

Interactive - use the internet links provided in the book to view online video while following the instruction taught in the book!

Details include:
Translation of Som Bo Gin (forward, arrow, scissors), Variance in Som Bo Gin training among Lam Sang's disciples, Speculation about Som Bo Gin, No Kwongsai Mantis Som Bo Gin in China, The meaning of Som Bo Gin, Som Bo Gin - nothing mysterious, The beginning and end of Southern Praying Mantis, Solo training, Paired training, Whole body power, Physical traits, Body weapons, Hakka Mantis posture, Footwork, Deep roots-iron steps, Forward momentum, Centerline theory, Bridge-range-distance, Frightening Spring Power, Contact-control-strike, Mantis summarized in three, Individual skills in Som Bo Gin two man; Call to mind drill, Unique hand and foot skills in Som Bo Gin Two Man, Bong Pun Shu, Yin Yang Sao, Bot Hop Shu, Mantis traps, Target Practice, Side to side steps, Lateral spins, Monkey step and kick, Step by step instructional photographs of Som Bo Gin Two Man form, Step by step breakdown of Som Bo Gin Two Man form in three lines and sixty postures A and B sides, Hakka Mantis history, a gallery of Louie Jack Man Sifu and RDH long form photographs, and more.

Book Specs
- Interactive www
- Hardcover
- Full color
- 250+ photographs
- 128 pages

Available at Amazon, Barnes and Noble, and other fine booksellers! Search Keywords - Southern Mantis Press

Our Family of Hakka Mantis Websites

Visit and Enjoy! Informational, Educational, Instructive

www.SouthernMantisPress.com

A ten year ongoing research in China
of the origins, history and practices of Southern Mantis!

Dedicated to the late Wong
Yuk Kong Sifu in China!
chinamantis.com

The Bamboo Temple Association
is a mutual aid fraternity. Join us
and become a member, School,
Branch or Study Group today!
Dedicated to the late Lam Sang
Sifu's teaching in the USA.
bambootemple.com
bambootemple-chicago.com
btcba.com

These sites reveal many China
Kwongsai Mantis Sifu who have
heretofore remained silent about
the teaching of Kwongsai
Dragon Tiger Mountain Bamboo Forest Temple Mantis and
outlines the lineage of Hakka Mantis as stated in China.
kwongsaimantis.com
somdotmantis.com

This site details the complete history of Chu Gar Gao Hakka
Praying Mantis as descended from the late Lao Sui in Hong Kong
and Hui Yang (Wai Yearn), China. (con't)

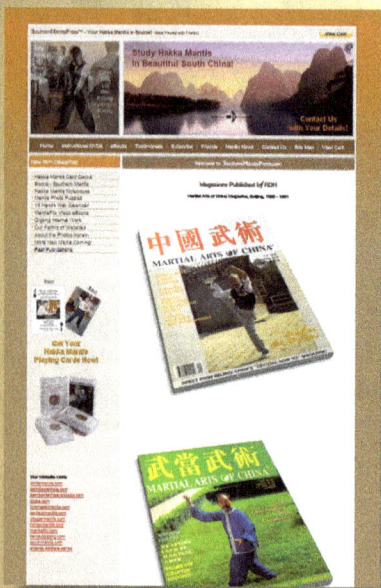

Resources

(con't) Dedicated to the late Cheng Wan Sifu who passed in 2009.
chugarmantis.com

This site is dedicated to the late Xu Fat Chun Sifu and speaks of the history of Iron Ox Hakka Praying Mantis in Pingdi Town, Guangdong, China.
ironoxmantis.com

Historical Hakka Mantis Flix! Some 60+ years of Hakka Southern Praying Mantis Kungfu movies and events in video eBooks!
mantisflix.com

Our dedicated South Mantis Tube. We have several hundreds of hours of videos in our Hakka Mantis archives dating back to 1950 in China that we hope to share with you! Feel free to share. Upload your Southern Mantis or Hakka video now!
southmantis.com

Genuine Internal Work - the original 11 month correspondence course of Tien Tao Qigong.
tientaoqigong.com

Ancient Methods to achieve vitality and a healthier well-being! The Oriental Secrets Series of Qigong.
oss.tientaoqigong.com

And visit our daily YouTube feed of only Southern Praying Mantis videos!
chinamantis.com/youtube

And our YouTube channel:
youtube.com/chinamantissurvey

Southern Mantis Instructional Playing Cards

Kwongsai Mantis
18 Buddha Hands

Card Backs: Various Sifu of Lam Sang's generations in multiple postures

Card Fronts: Two man application photos, Text instruction, Instructive maxims

Includes the 18 Buddha Hands and more of Kwongsai Hakka Mantis

For ♣ A
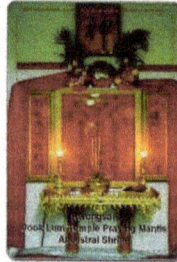

For ♦ A
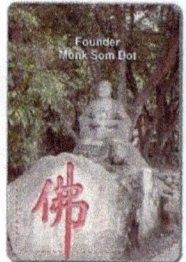

For ♠ 2
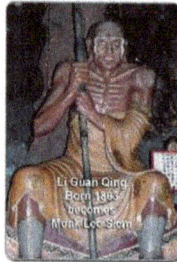

For ♥ 2
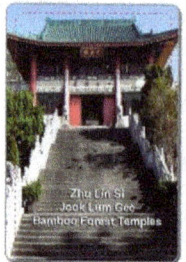

Key Benefits
of our Card Decks

- 54 Cards with Hakka Mantis
- Customized Front and Back
- Full Vibrant Color!
- Instructional
- Educational
- Informative
- Rare and Exclusive Content and Photographs
- Entertaining - Play Hakka Mantis Cards with your friends

Front
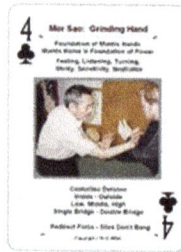

Back
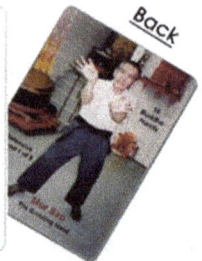

Front
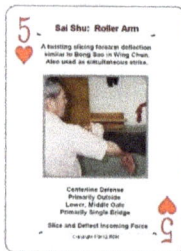

Back
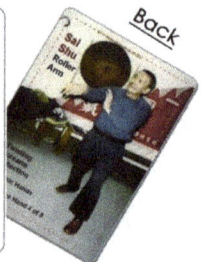

MantisFlix™ Video eBooks

60 Years of Southern Mantis Movies and Events!

Wong Fei Hong and the Jook Lum Temple

Volume 1001 - Hong Kong 1954

B/W Classic Movie Exclusive! 100,000 plus clip previews on YouTube. Get your full copy now!

Kwongsai Mantis Celebration

Volume 1002 - Pingshan Town, Guangdong, China

Late Sifu Wong Yuk Kong Kwongsai Jook Lum Clan 35th Anniversary Celebration, circa 2003.

Hakka Boxing Collection One
Volume 1003 - A rare collection of Hakka Boxing.

Hakka Boxing Collection Two
Volume 1004 - A second rare collection of Hakka Boxing.

Chu Gar Cheng Wan Celebration
Volume 1005 - Join the 1989 Cheng Wan Chu Gar Mantis Celebration in Hong Kong! Cheng Wan Sifu was the inheritor of Chu Gar descended from Lao Sui.

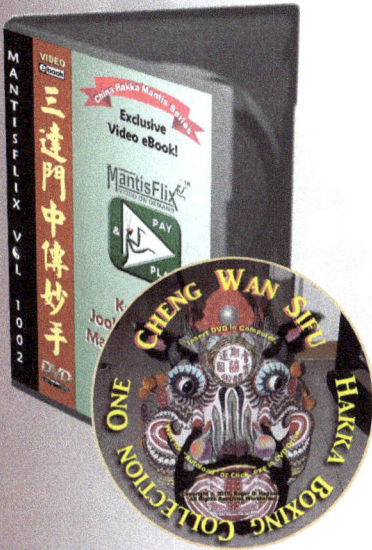

View and Enjoy Video Previews Online:
www.MantisFlix.com

ChinaMantis.com   Instructional DVDs

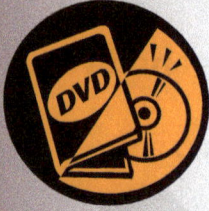

Jook Lum Temple Mantis
Step by Step Instruction
in 18 Volumes

Year One Training

Volume One: Fundamentals; The Most Important
Volume Two: Phoenix Eye Fist Attacking / Stepping
Volume Three: Centerline Defense
Volume Four: One, Three & Nine Step Attack / Defense
Volume Five: Centerline Sticky Hand Training
Volume Six: Same Hand / Opposite Hand Attacks
Volume Seven: Sai Shu, Sik Shu, Jik (Chun) Shu
Volume Eight: Gow Choy; Hammer Fist-Internal Strength
Volume Nine: Footwork in Southern Praying Mantis
Volume 10:   Chi Sao Sticky Hands and Passoffs

Advanced Two Man Forms—Year Two and Three

Available by request. Prerequisite Volumes 1– 10.
Volume 11: Loose Hands One
Volume 12: Som Bo Gin
Volume 13: Second Loose Hands
Volume 14: 108 Subset
Volume 15: Um Hon One
Volume 16: Um Hon Two
Volume 17: Mui Fa Plum Flower
Volume 18: Eighteen Buddha Hands

All 8 two man forms must be trained as one continuous set on both A - B sides.

DVD Descriptions and Video Clips

http://www.southernmantispress.com/instructional-dvds.htm

Summary Year One

http://www.chinamantis.com/first-year-training.htm

Join a School or Start a Study Group

Hakka "Southern" Praying Mantis Kungfu
Bamboo Temple Chinese Benevolent Association
Hong Kong Chu Gar Mantis Martial Art Association

Roger D. Hagood, Standing Chairman
Hong Kong, Shenzhen, China
rdh@chinamantis.com

USA

Crystal Lake, Illinois School
Richard Lee Gamboa
USA Chief Instructor
Phone: (847) 458-2080
Mantis@ActionKungFu.com

Los Angeles, CA School
John Brown
Phone: (510) 423 1615
Tonglong108@gmail.com

Huntsville - North AL, Branch
Slade White
256-694-0949
slade@sladewhite.com

Indiana, USA Branch
Dave Marshall
812-709-0827
ictdave@aol.com

Washington DC Study Group
Eric Lewis
240-552-1338
jooklumspm@gmail.com

Weslaco, TX Study Group
David Garcia
(956) 472-0254
garciads1@gmail.com

INT'L

Taipei, Taiwan Branch
Dr. Han Chih Lu
simonclh@gmail.com

London, Ontario, Canada Branch
Mike Shaw
Phone 519-852-2174
mantismike@start.ca

Düsseldorf, Germany Branch
Erik Irsch
eirsch@yahoo.de

Lima, Peru Study Group
Guillermo E. Talavera
getalavera@hotmail.com

Lugansk, Ukraine Study Group
Andrew V. Potapov
mantis_ukraine@ukr.net

Like minded people that have a sincere interest to study Southern Praying Mantis together and are following the Instructional DVDs may start a Study Group.
Become a group leader today!

RDH: Publisher's Page
Plum Flower Mantis; South Korea; 1976-1978

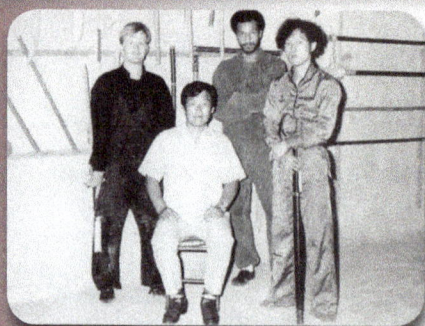

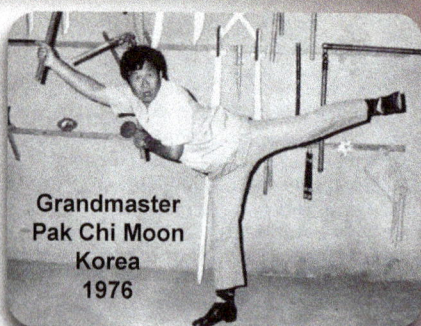

Grandmaster
Pak Chi Moon
Korea
1976

Grandteacher Pak Chi Moon seated. RDH in black. Brothers Cho & Drake

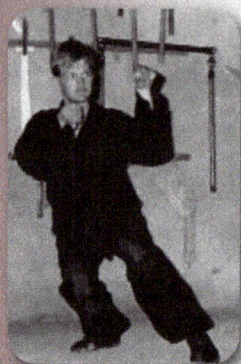

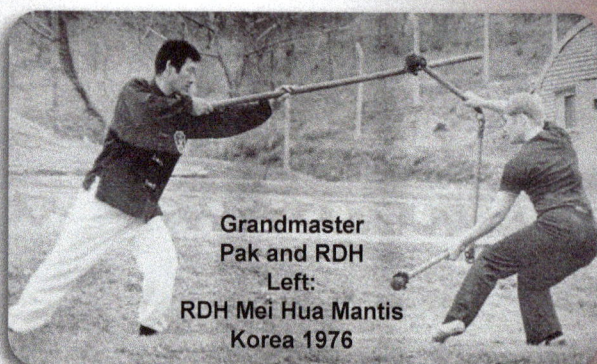

Grandmaster
Pak and RDH
Left:
RDH Mei Hua Mantis
Korea 1976

RDH's first Black Belt rank was Hawaiian Kenpo, 1972, after 5 years training

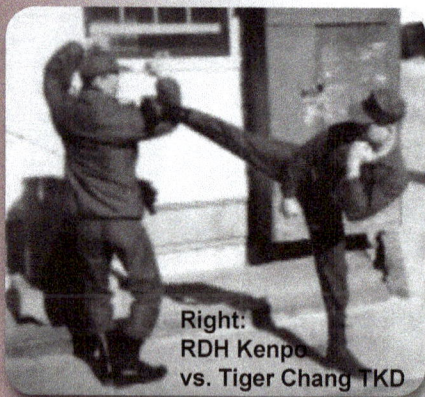

Right:
RDH Kenpo
vs. Tiger Chang TKD

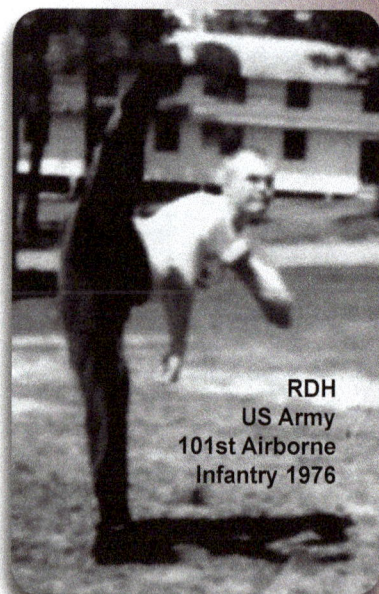

RDH
US Army
101st Airborne
Infantry 1976

RDH has concentrated on martial arts training since 1967 and specialized in Southern Praying Mantis from 1980 onward. Since 2002, he has lived in China where he teaches Hakka Mantis.

RDH has been featured in various international publications and television shows from China and Taiwan to Mexico and the USA.

The two photos right are reproduced from a 1989 USA newspaper article entitled, *"RDH - Modern Renaissance Man"*

The *RDH: Publisher's Page* left is reproduced from *Grandmasters* newsstand magazine circa 1990.

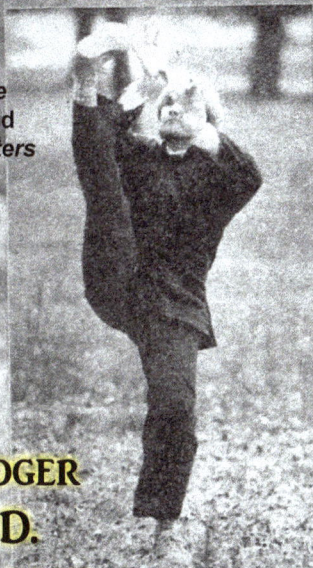

ROGER D. HAGOOD

RDH Bio

Welcome to visit the Publisher!

Your email correspondence is welcome and do visit and study Hakka Southern Praying Mantis with me in beautiful sunny south China! I am an Author, Publisher and Producer of eBooks, books, journals, videos and 7 International martial arts newsstand magazines in 15 countries with 45 years in training and teaching martial arts and some 20 years living in China and Asia!

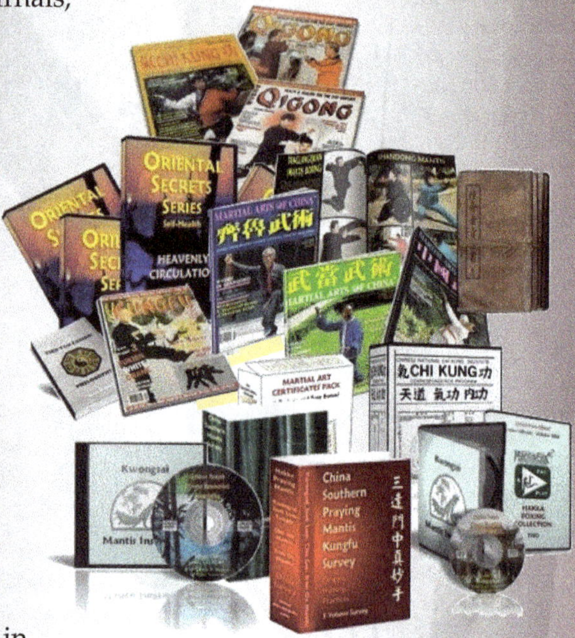

Currently residing in beautiful sunny south China for the last 11 years where I teach Southern Praying Mantis. Join my class in Guangdong today!

RDH
Pingshan Town
Winter, 2012

More Bio:
http://www.chinamantis.com/roger-d.-hagood.htm
Email:
rdh@chinamantis.com

116

Study Hakka Mantis and Unicorn in China

Study in Beautiful South China!

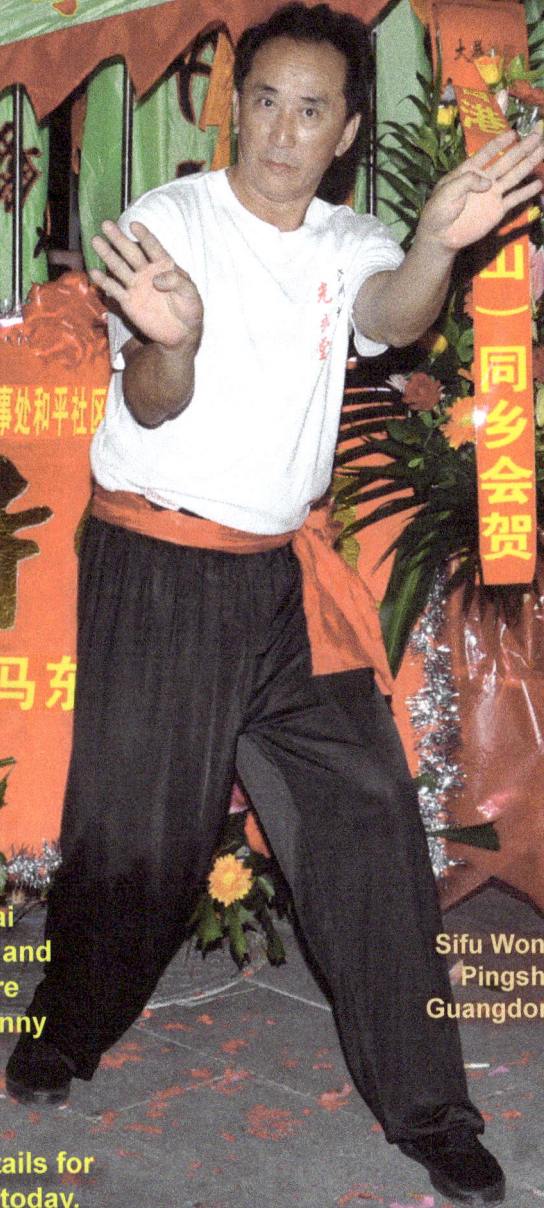

Train Kwongsai Hakka Mantis and Unicorn Culture in beautiful sunny South China!

Sifu Wong Yu Hua Pingshan Town, Guangdong, China

Email your details for consideration today.
rdh@chinamantis.com

117

Six Internals

- **SKILLFULNESS:** movements should be varied, unexpected and flexible

- **TACTFULNESS:** control the opponent using his strength

- **BOLDNESS:** strike immediately without resolve

- **SWIFTNESS:** use visible fists to strike invisible blows

- **FIERCENESS:** attack the vital parts with intent

- **PRACTICAL:** train attack and defense; nothing for show

WUDANG MOUNTAIN

Northwestern Hubei Province, China

Home of Internal Work

The Wudang School was founded by Zhang Sanfeng, a Taoist in the early Ming Dynasty (1368-1644) reputed for his intelligence and erudition. During his 23 year stay in the Wudang Mountains, he learned martial arts and integrated them with internal organ and breath control.

武當山